ABC OF PALLIATIVE CARE

Second Edition

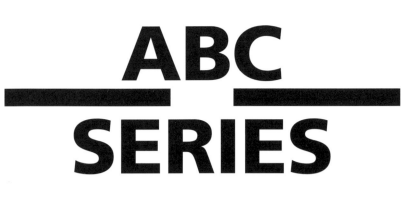

ABC SERIES

- More than 40 titles supplying quick and dependable answers to your most common questions on a range of topics in all the major specialties

- Each title reflects the high standards of the BMJ, which peer reviews and serialises the articles before being published in this great series of books

- A consistent format keeps the books easy to use, with pages laid out in two columns and a heavily illustrated 'slide show' accompanying the text

- Key features such as photographs, graphs and diagnostic images help pull out the fundamental points

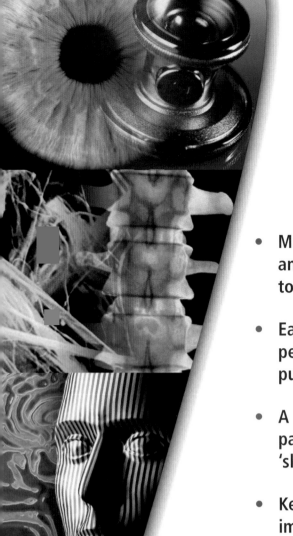

ABC OF **EMERGENCY RADIOLOGY** SECOND EDITION
Edited by Otto Chan

ABC OF **HEALTH INFORMATICS**
Frank Sullivan and Jeremy C Wyatt

ABC OF **CONFLICT AND DISASTER**
Edited by Anthony D Redmond, Peter F Mahoney, James M Ryan and Cara's Macnab
Foreword by Lord David Owen

ABC OF **WOUND HEALING**
Edited by Joseph E Grey and Keith G Harding

Blackwell Publishing
Partnerships in learning, research and professional practice

For further information on the whole of the ABC series, please visit

www.bmjbooks.com

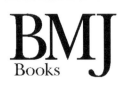

BMJ Books

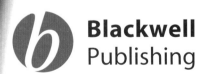

ABC OF PALLIATIVE CARE

Second Edition

Edited by

MARIE FALLON
St Columba's Hospice Chair of Palliative Medicine,
University of Edinburgh, Edinburgh

and

GEOFFREY HANKS
Professor of Palliative Medicine, University of Bristol, Bristol

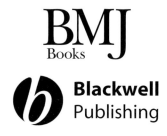

BMJ
Books

Blackwell
Publishing

Blackwell Publishing, Inc., 350 Main Street, Malden, Massachusetts 02148-5020, USA
Blackwell Publishing Ltd, 9600 Garsington Road, Oxford OX4 2DQ, UK
Blackwell Publishing Asia Pty Ltd, 550 Swanston Street, Carlton, Victoria 3053, Australia

First published 1998
Second edition 2006

1 2006

Library of Congress Cataloging-in-Publication Data
ABC of palliative care/edited by Marie Fallon and Geoffrey Hanks. — 2nd ed.
      p. ; cm.
   "BMJ Books."
   Includes bibliographical references and index.
   ISBN-13: 978-1-4051-3079-0 (alk.paper)
   ISBN-10: 1-4051-3079-2 (alk.paper)
  1. Palliative treatment. 2. Terminal care. I. Fallon, Marie. II. Hanks, Geoffrey W. C.
   [DNLM: 1. Palliative Care—methods. 2. Palliative Care—psychology. 3. Terminal Care.
WB 310 A134 2006]

   R726.8.A23 2006
   616′.029—dc22

                                                                                              2006009883

ISBN-13: 978 1 4051 3079 0
ISBN-10: 1 4051 3079 2

A catalogue record for this title is available from the British Library

Cover image is courtesy of John Cole/Science Photo Library

Set in 9/11 pt by Newgen Imaging Systems (P) Ltd, Chennai, India
Printed and bound in Singapore by COS Printers Pte Ltd

Commissioning Editor: Eleanor Lines
Development Editors: Sally Carter, Nick Morgan
Senior Technical Editor: Barbara Squire
Editorial Assistants: Francesca Naish, Victoria Pittman
Production Controller: Debbie Wyer

For further information on Blackwell Publishing, visit our website:
http://www.blackwellpublishing.com

Contents

Contributors

James Adam
Consultant in Palliative Medicine, Hunter's Hill Marie Curie Centre, Glasgow

Julia Addington-Hall
Professor of End-of-Life Care, University of Southampton

Jeremy Bagg
Professor of Clinical Microbiology, Glasgow Dental Hospital and School, Glasgow

Matthew Barber
Consultant Surgeon, Edinburgh Cancer Centre, Edinburgh

Gian Borasio
Interdisciplinary Palliative Care Unit, Department of Neurology, Munich, Germany

Eduardo Bruera
Professor of Oncology, UT MD Anderson Cancer Center, Houston, Texas, USA

Joanna Chambers
Consultant in Oncology and Palliative Medicine, Southmead Hospital, Bristol

Nathan Cherny
Director of Cancer Pain and Palliative Medicine, Share Zedek Medical Center, Jerusalem, Israel

Lesley Colvin
Consultant Anaesthetist, Department of Clinical Neurosciences, Western General Hospital, Edinburgh

Andrew Davies
Consultant in Palliative Medicine, Royal Marsden Hospital, London

Carol Davis
Consultant in Palliative Medicine, Moorgreen Hospital, Southampton

Francis Dunn
Consultant Cardiologist, Stobhill Hospital, Glasgow

Stephen Falk
Consultant in Clinical Oncology, Bristol Haematology and Oncology Centre, Bristol

Marie Fallon
St Columba's Hospice Chair of Palliative Medicine, University of Edinburgh, Edinburgh

Kenneth Fearon
Professor of Surgical Oncology, University of Edinburgh, Edinburgh

Karen Forbes
Macmillan Professorial Teaching Fellow in Palliative Medicine, Department of Palliative Medicine, Bristol Haematology and Oncology Centre, Bristol

Rob George
Consultant in Palliative Medicine, Meadow House Hospice, Middlesex

Ann Goldman
CLIC Consultant in Palliative Care, Great Ormond Street Hospital for Children, London

Debra Gordon
Clinical Nurse Specialist in Palliative Medicine, Western General Hospital, Edinburgh

Geoffrey Hanks
Professor of Palliative Medicine, University of Bristol, Bristol

David Jeffrey
Consultant in Palliative Medicine, Borders General Hospital, Scotland

Michelle Kohn
Complementary Therapy Adviser, London

Mari Lloyd-Williams
Professor, Academic Palliative and Supportive Care Studies Group, Division of Primary Care, University of Liverpool, Liverpool

Lorna McGoldrick
Clinical Nurse Specialist, Palliative Care, Western General Hospital, Edinburgh

Jane Maher
Consultant Oncologist, Mount Vernon Cancer Centre, Middlesex

Kathryn Mannix
Consultant in Palliative Medicine, Marie Curie Centre, Newcastle-upon-Tyne

Balfour Mount
Professor of Palliative Medicine, Department of Oncology, McGill University, Montreal, Quebec, Canada

Gillian Percy
Clinical Specialist Physiotherapist, Moorgreen Hospital, Southampton

Amanda Ramirez
Professor of Liaison Psychiatry, Institute of Psychiatry, King's College, London

Colette Reid
Research Fellow in Palliative Medicine, Bristol Haematology and Oncology Centre, Bristol

Marilyn Relf
Head of Education, Churchill Hospital, Oxford

Carla Ripamonti
Palliative Care Physician, National Cancer Institute of Milan, Milan, Italy

Nigel Sykes
Medical Director, St Christopher's Hospice, Sydenham, London

Keri Thomas
Macmillan GP facilitator, Shrewsbury

Raymond Voltz
Consultant Neurologist, Institute for Clinical Neuroimmunology, Munich, Germany

Roger Woodruff
Director of Palliative Care, Austin and Repatriation Centre, Heidelberg, Victoria, Australia

Foreword

It is almost impossible for a health care professional to avoid being called upon to care for people getting frailer as life ebbs away, to care for them at their dying and to have to help and support their loved ones afterwards. Who can be insensitive to their pain, their breathlessness, their weakness and their fears? Who can forget how helpless they have felt at these times, how lost for words, how unskilled and unprepared. Doctors and nurses, whether generalist or specialist, can no more avoid these professional and personal challenges than they can deny or avoid death itself.

Palliative care – "*the care of patients with active, progressive, advanced disease where the prognosis is short and the focus of care is the quality of life*" – is a basic human right, not a luxury for the few. Its principles are not peculiar to the care of the dying but are the integral features of all good clinical care – freedom from pain and the alleviation so far as is possible, of all physical, psychosocial and spiritual suffering; the preservation of dignity; the utmost respect for honesty in all our dealings with these patients and their relatives.

The emergence in 1987 of palliative care as a medical sub-specialty (mentioned in the Preface to the first edition of this book) has brought about improvements in care, research, professional education and training, and in the understanding by the public and the politicians of what needs to be done and what can be done for those at the loneliest time on their life journey. It has also had a downside. Many have come to suspect that providing palliative care requires unique people to do justice to this demanding work, unique skills to do it well, and more time than today's doctors and nurses ever have. So easy is it to phone a palliative care specialist whether working in a hospital, a specialist unit or in the community, and get advice or an admission that some are leaving the palliative care of their patients to them. In fact only about 10% of terminally ill patients have problems so rare or so complex that specialist expertise is needed. All the others can be cared for by non-specialists if they learn the principles of palliative care, if they develop the right attitude to it, if they are willing to share themselves as well as their therapeutic skills... and if they study this book. One thing is undeniable – no-one is born with a built-in ability to provide excellent care. It has to be learnt from a book such as this, and hopefully from watching others with more experience, but that is a luxury some never have.

In situations where too often the knee-jerk response can be "there is no more we can do", the reader will find that there is always a means of helping and of caring. It may be pharmacological or psychological, nursing or physiotherapy, occupational therapy, music or art therapy, or complementary medicine. Often it may be no more, no less than enabling patients to open their hearts in that atmosphere of safety created by the doctor or nurse who has learned to be honest, and is humble enough to listen and to learn.

The reader will be surprised at how richly rewarding palliative care can be; how surprisingly often terminally ill patients speak of the sense of safety they feel when suffering has been relieved and they know everyone is being honest with them and the loved ones they will leave behind. This can happen anywhere – in a hospital, in a hospice, in a nursing home or in someone's home.

This excellent book produced by editors and contributors with international reputations deserves to be read by every doctor and nurse who will ever offer palliative care – and that means most of us!

Derek Doyle
Retired consultant in palliative medicine
Vice President, National Council for Palliative Care
Founding Member and Adviser,
International Association for Hospice and Palliative Care

1 The principles of palliative care

Balfour Mount, Geoffrey Hanks, Lorna McGoldrick

Components of palliative care

Palliative care is recognised by individualised, holistic models of care, delivered carefully, sensitively, ethically, and therapeutically by using skilled communication with attention to detail, meticulous assessment, and advancing knowledge.

Wherever palliative care is used, its core ingredient is the quality of presence that the caregiver brings to the patient, a way of caring that enables discernment of the ongoing needs of the patient and family as they evolve and emphasises being alongside them. The focus is on all that is still possible in this time of multiple losses, the patient's and family's quest for meaning, and sustaining their experience of connectedness as they adapt to the challenges of the moment.

The term "palliative care" implies a personalised form of health care. It extends the healthcare professional's mandate beyond the biomedical model to the wider horizon necessary if one is to attend to suffering as well as the biology of disease, caring as well as curing, quality of life as well as quantity of life. The patient and family or significant others are taken together as the unit of care in assessment of needs related to illness. The aim of palliative care is to support optimal quality of life and to foster healing—that is, a shift in response towards an experience of *integrity* and wholeness on the continuum of the quality of life.

Beyond the physical

Meticulous attention to the alleviation of symptoms is the foundation of care of the whole person. Important psychosocial and spiritual concerns may be eclipsed by the presence of uncontrolled pain, nausea, constipation, and the other symptoms of advanced disease. Optimal treatment demands careful assessment of the multiple contributory factors to each symptom. If increasing doses of opioid are prescribed in response to pain that is escalating due to unrecognised existential anguish, the result will be persistent pain, opioid toxicity, and ongoing distress for the patient, family, and caregivers. If we are body, mind, and spirit, those domains are inseparable and interdependent. Thoughtful assessment of each complaint should be considered in the context of the patient's total suffering; therefore thoughtful assessment is mandatory.

Not just symptom control

Control of symptoms in palliative care commonly involves the concurrent use of six to eight or more medications. The goal is consistently to prevent rather than treat symptoms. Effective management depends on frequent adjustment to consistently sustain the minimal effective doses of medication and an emphasis on skilled nursing care as well as the use of the complementary skills of an interdisciplinary team experienced in end of life care.

Laboratory investigations—and even such non-invasive routines as monitoring blood pressure, pulse, and temperature—are undertaken only if doing so may lead to interventions that will enhance the quality of life.

Palliative care is founded on a philosophy that promotes sensitivity to cultural, religious, sexual, and other defining perspectives from the patient's point of view; the intent to meet patients where they are rather than where the caregivers feel they should be; sensitivity to the determinants of coping, particularly concerning major existential challenges for the

> Palliative care is the approach that improves the quality of life of patients and their families facing the problems associated with life threatening illness, through the prevention and relief of suffering by means of early identification and impeccable assessment and treatment of pain and other problems, physical, psychosocial, and spiritual (World Health Organization, 2005)

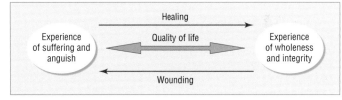

The quality of life continuum

Palliative care: selected philosophical perspectives and assumptions

- Nothing matters more than the bowels (Cecily Saunders)
- Humanise, personalise, de-institutionalise
- Clinical care grounded in qualitative and quantitative inquiry
- Experience of illness viewed as a narrative: relational, meaningful, filled with potential
- Assist progressive understanding of reality at a rate acceptable to the patient
- "Reality" as illusion; subjectivity of experience; acknowledgment of mystery
- Quiet efficiency, not hustle and bustle
- Focus on quality of living in the present moment, not death
- Accompaniment: empathic presence to the other in the moment
- Team: led by the patient; egalitarian rather than hierarchical
- Environment: centred on the patient, welcoming, peaceful
- Uniqueness, limitations, defences of the patient/family
- Healing of psyche: an innate potential
- Potential for adaptation, integration, reconciliation, transcendence
- Importance of compassion, celebration, community, paradox, humour
- With unresolved symptoms, "Review! Review! Review!" (Robert Twycross)

patient, family, and caregivers (death; isolation; freedom—the absence of external structure; meaning); attention to the meaning of the illness for the patient, family, and caregivers; and attention to the need for relating to people in an empathic way.

Application

The early successes of hospice care in alleviating the suffering of patients with cancer and those with motor neurone disease and some other neurodegenerative diseases at the end of life has led now to broad agreement concerning the relevance of palliative care across the spectrum of disease and healthcare settings.

Care delivery

Considerations in the provision of palliative care include a seamless continuity of care appropriate to the needs of the patient and the family, with options that include home care; chronic inpatient care; acute, specialised inpatient (tertiary) care; consultation services available for those still receiving treatment to modify the disease; day care with resources for multidisciplinary assessment; bereavement support for those at risk of a complicated grief reaction.

Specialist role

General palliative care is practiced widely in specialties other than palliative care. Multiprofessional teams who work full time in palliative care, and are trained beyond the basic level, deliver specialist palliative care. They aim to care for those patients and carers who have complex physical, psychosocial, or spiritual needs that are difficult to manage. Their role is primarily about advice, support, and education when they work alongside other specialties. Hospices and hospice wards have more direct management of patients and carers in an inpatient setting. Role modelling, service development in line with local, national, and WHO guidelines, education, and research are further components of the role.

Multidisciplinary teams

Caring for patients and carers at a difficult time is synonymous with palliative care. Each patient and carer will require a unique and individualised approach to incorporate all their biopsychosocial and spiritual needs. There cannot be a universal optimum model for the delivery of care; adaptability and flexibility is paramount, and this is an increasing challenge in today's healthcare systems.

A single profession, like a single model of care, can only fail to meet the holistic fluctuating needs of patients and carers. The knowledge and skill of many professions—medical, nursing, pharmacy, social work, physiotherapy, occupational therapy, and chaplaincy—held together by endless communication and teamwork is vital.

Future challenges

New and evolving challenges in palliative care are emerging as patients live longer with improved palliative tumoricidal treatments. Symptoms that are difficult to control and are chronically debilitating test the resilience and resources of weary patients, carers, and providers of health care. Education and robust multiprofessional support are necessary to equip those working in palliative care with the sustainable resilience

---

Initial hospice programmes:
predominantly oncology and selected neurodegenerative diseases

| Life prolonging therapy | Palliative care |

Palliative care relevance, current view:
all end stage diseases and clinical settings

| Life prolonging therapy | Palliative care |

Changes in allocation of resources with the development of palliative care

---

Palliative care
- Affirms life and regards dying as a normal practice
- Neither hastens nor postpones death
- Provides relief from pain and other distressing symptoms
- Integrates the psychological and spiritual aspects of care
- Offers a support system to help patients live as actively as possible until death
- Offers a support system to help the families of patients cope during the patient's illnesses and in their own bereavement

---

Essential components of palliative care
- Control of symptoms
- Effective communication
- Rehabilitation
- Continuity of care
- Terminal care
- Support in bereavement
- Education
- Research

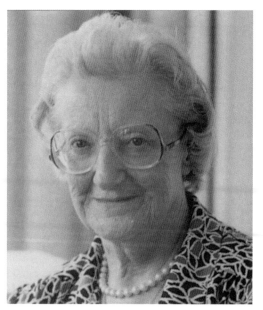

Dame Cecily Saunders, founder of St Christopher's Hospice (reproduced with permission)

demanded by an unwavering quality of presence that continues to effectively focus on quality of life and care and attend to suffering of patients with longer and more difficult experiences.

Without research, advances in the science of control of symptoms and quality of care will stagnate and palliative care will cease to meet the future needs of patients with advanced life threatening illnesses and their carers. Though there are numerous epidemiological surveys outlining problems, few researchers do good quality interventional studies or try to extend knowledge through collaboration with basic science. More collaborative research involving basic science and other appropriate specialties is needed urgently.

The late Dame Cecily Saunders and her vision of combining optimum care, observation, and appropriate research established the essential ingredients of modern palliative care; this should remain our basis for the future.

Further reading

- Cassell EJ. *The nature of suffering and the goals of medicine.* 2nd ed. New York: Oxford University Press, 2004.
- Doyle D, Hanks GW, Cherny N, Calman K, eds. *The Oxford textbook of palliative medicine.* 3rd ed. Oxford: Oxford University Press, 2004.
- Halpern J. *From detached concern to empathy: humanizing medical practice.* New York: Oxford University Press, 2001.
- Kearney M. *A place of healing: working with suffering in living and dying.* Oxford: Oxford University Press, 2000.
- Saunders C, Sykes N. *The management of terminal disease.* 3rd ed. London: Edward Arnold, 1993.
- Yalom ID. *Existential psychotherapy.* New York: Basic Books, 1980.

2   The principles of control of cancer pain

Marie Fallon, Geoffrey Hanks, Nathan Cherny

Pain is a complex phenomenon which is the subjective endpoint of a variety of physical and non-physical factors. For most patients, physical pain is only one of several symptoms of cancer. Relief of pain should therefore be seen as part of a comprehensive pattern of care encompassing the physical, psychological, social, and spiritual aspects of suffering. Physical aspects of pain cannot be treated in isolation from other aspects, nor can patients' anxieties be effectively addressed when patients are suffering physically. The various components must be addressed simultaneously.

Our understanding of the basic mechanisms of pain has improved considerably over the past few years. This understanding has included a greater appreciation of the relationship between the physical injury, pain pathways, and our emotional processing of this information; these factors are interlinked in the nervous system, rather than working in parallel. We now understand from basic science more of the mechanisms of total pain than ever before. It is clear that anxiety, fear, and sleeplessness feed into the limbic system and cortex. In turn, the brain talks back to the spinal cord modifying pain input at spinal levels. This then feeds back to the brain and a loop is established.

Mood disturbance is common in patients with uncontrolled cancer pain and may need specific management, however, sometimes it will improve dramatically with effective resolution of pain. Hence the first principle of managing cancer pain is an adequate and full assessment of the cause of the pain, bearing in mind that most patients have more than one pain. With effective assessment and a systematic approach to the choice of analgesics using the WHO's three step analgesic ladder, over 80% of cancer pain can be controlled with the use of inexpensive drugs that can be self administered by mouth at regular intervals.

The WHO analgesic ladder

The analgesic ladder remains the mainstay of our approach to analgesia, though this was never designed for use in isolation. Surgery, radiotherapy, and appropriate tumoricidal treatments will have an important role in some patients, as will non-drug treatments. A combined approach can lead to optimum analgesia with minimum side effects.

Analgesic drugs do, however, remain key in managing cancer pain. The choice of drug should be based on the severity of the pain, not the stage of disease. Drugs should be administered in standard doses at regular intervals in a stepwise fashion. If a non-opioid or, in turn, an opioid for moderate pain is not sufficient, an opioid for severe pain should be used.

When a non-opioid drug is used with an opioid for moderate pain, many patients find combination formulations more convenient to use. Care must be taken with the dose of each drug in the formulation; some combinations of codeine or dihydrocodeine with aspirin or paracetamol (including co-codamol and co-dydramol) contain subtherapeutic doses of the opioid. The decision to use an opioid for severe pain should be based on severity of pain and not on prognosis.

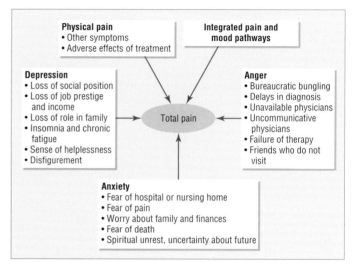

Factors affecting patient's perceptions of pain (adapted from Twycross RG, Lack SA, *Therapeutics in terminal disease*, London: Pitman, 1984)

Analgesic drugs commonly recommended for cancer pain

Mild pain
- Aspirin 600 mg four times a day
- Paracetamol 1 g four times a day

Moderate pain
- Codeine 60 mg (plus non-opioid drug) four times a day

Severe pain
- Morphine 5–10 mg (starting dose) every four hours

Non-drug treatments used in management of cancer pain
- TENS (transcutaneous electrical nerve stimulation)
- Physiotherapy
- Acupuncture
- Relaxation therapy

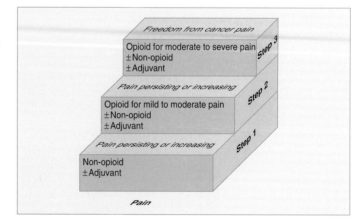

WHO analgesic ladder (adapted from WHO's *Cancer pain relief and palliative care* technical report series 804)

Adjuvant analgesics

Adjuvant analgesic drugs may be usefully added at any stage. An adjuvant analgesic is a drug whose primary indication is for something other than pain but that has an analgesic effect in some painful conditions. Examples are corticosteroids, non-steroidal anti-inflammatory drugs, tricyclic antidepressants, anticonvulsants, and some antiarrhythmic drugs.

Tricyclic antidepressants and anticonvulsants

Tricyclic antidepressants are effective in relieving neuropathic pain. There are no significant differences in efficacy between the different tricyclic antidepressants, though unfortunately, side effects often limit their use. While the evidence for venlafaxine is less strong, its use can be justified, particularly in patients with both neuropathic pain and low mood. There is a lack of high level evidence of the efficacy of selective serotonin reuptake inhibitors (SSRIs) for treating neuropathic pain.

The anticonvulsants carbamazepine, phenytoin, sodium valproate, clonazepam, gabapentin, and pregabalin are effective in treating neuropathic pain. Benefit is independent of the characteristics of the pain. Gabapentin and pregabalin are licensed for treatment of neuropathic pain.

There is no measurable difference in the analgesic benefit of the two drug classes (tricyclic antidepressants or anticonvulsants) in neuropathic pain or in the number of patients needed to treat before a minor or major adverse effect occurs. Gabapentin and pregabalin, however, can have fewer side effects in many patients, though systematic examination of this is awaited in patients with cancer pain.

Patients with neuropathic pain should have a trial of a tricyclic antidepressant or venlafaxine or an anticonvulsant. The choice of drug should be based on relative contraindications, possible drug interactions, and risk of side effects for each patient. Antidepressants and anticonvulsants may occasionally be prescribed simultaneously, though it is good clinical practice to introduce only one drug at a time.

Opioid analgesics for severe pain

Morphine is the most commonly used opioid in this group. When possible, it should be given by mouth, the dose tailored to each patient, and doses repeated at regular intervals so that the pain is prevented from returning. There is no arbitrary upper limit, but negative attitudes to using morphine still exist.

Dose titration—A normal release formulation of morphine (either elixir or tablet), with a rapid onset and short duration of action, is preferred for dose titration. The simplest method is to prescribe a regular four hourly dose but allow extra doses of the same size for "breakthrough pain" as often as necessary. After 24 or 48 hours, the daily requirements may be reassessed and the regular dose adjusted as necessary. This process is continued until pain relief is satisfactory. By this method, the many factors that contribute to the variability in dose are taken into account. These include the severity of the pain, the type of pain, the affective component of pain, and variation in pharmacokinetic parameters. The regular four hourly dose may range from 5–10 mg to ≥250 mg (or the equivalent in controlled release tablets). The dose is titrated against effect, though few patients need high doses—with most requiring <200 mg a day.

Maintenance dose—Patients with advancing disease and increasing pain may require continual adjustment of dose. For many patients, however, there is a period of stability during which the dose required remains unchanged or needs only small adjustments, and this may last for weeks or months or sometimes longer. Once pain is relieved, maintenance will be

Common adjuvant analgesics for cancer pain

Drugs	Indications
Non-steroidal anti-inflammatory drugs	Bone pain Soft tissue infiltration Hepatomegaly
Corticosteroids	Raised intracranial pressure Soft tissue infiltration Nerve compression Hepatomegaly
Antidepressants Anticonvulsants Antiarrhythmics	Nerve compression or infiltration Paraneoplastic neuropathies
Bisphosphonates	Bone pain

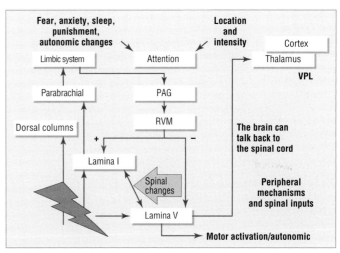

Integration of pain and emotion at higher centres. With permission from Professor A. Dickenson

> **The skilled use of morphine will confer benefit rather than harm, but many patients express fears, which should be discussed**

Opioid alternatives to morphine

- *Hydromorphone*—Titration is usually with hydromorphone normal release capsules; when pain is controlled, patients may convert to controlled release preparation. As it is about seven times stronger than morphine, care is needed with patients with no previous exposure to opioids
- *Oxycodone*—Can be up to 1.5 times stronger than morphine. Similar titration as morphine and hydromorphone
- *Methadone*—see chapter 3, Difficult pain
- *Fentanyl*—Self adhesive patches provide transcutaneous delivery of strong opioid. The patch is changed once every 72 hours. It is used with normal release morphine for breakthrough pain. It is suitable only for patients whose pain is stable because of the time required to titrate the dose upwards. It takes up to 24–48 hours before peak plasma concentrations are achieved
- *Buprenorphine*—Transdermal, as above, and may have advantages in patients with renal dysfunction
- *Diamorphine*, limited availability, is a semisynthetic derivative and a prodrug of morphine. Use of oral diamorphine is an inefficient way of delivering morphine to the body, but, for parenteral administration, its greater solubility confers an advantage over morphine
- *Pethidine* is a short acting opioid and not appropriate for the management of chronic pain

with a controlled release preparation of morphine. Controlled release morphine is available as a once daily preparation that remains effective for 24 hours or a twice daily preparation with effects that last 12 hours.

Alternative routes of administration

The rectal bioavailability of morphine is similar to its oral bioavailability, and it is available in suppository form. The rectal route may be appropriate for patients unable to take drugs by mouth, and the same dose as that taken orally should be given every four hours.

For many patients, however, it may be more convenient to convert directly to a subcutaneous infusion of opioid via an infusion device such as a portable, pocket sized, syringe driver. This simple technique allows continuous infusion of opioid analgesics in patients unable to take drugs by mouth. The relative potency of opioids is increased when they are given parenterally: the oral dose of morphine should be halved to get the equianalgesic dose of subcutaneous morphine and halved or divided by three for subcutaneous diamorphine, depending on the clinical situation.

Rarely, patients may require intravenous administration, which can be appropriate for those with an indwelling central line, particularly children.

Which opioid for cancer pain?

Comparative trials of opioids in cancer pain are extremely difficult to perform and do not always answer our questions because of the complexity of the populations studied. A tension exists between the need to have good quality randomised controlled trials to provide evidence for pharmacotherapy of cancer pain and the appropriateness and complexities of such trials in patients with advanced cancer.

No strong evidence supports the superiority of one opioid over another. However, the balance between analgesia and side effects varies among opioids because of factors such as pharmacokinetic profiles, routes of administration, and genetic variability in opioid responses.

The transdermal route, which can be used with fentanyl or transdermal buprenorphine, can be useful in patients with swallowing difficulties. Oxycodone or hydromorphone may provide an alternative to morphine if hallucinations or disturbed sleep are troublesome.

Any opioid can accumulate in patients with renal dysfunction. It is clear we do not fully understand the various metabolites from different opioids. Care should always be taken and in such patients opioid doses should generally be lower than normal, with increased intervals between doses, or even administered on an "as required" basis. It is usually acceptable to consider use of drugs such as fentanyl, alfentanil, hydromorphone, and buprenorphine.

Tolerance, addiction, and physical dependence

Tolerance to opioids is rarely seen in the clinical practice of managing cancer pain. Requirements for increasing doses of morphine can usually be explained by progressive disease rather than pharmacological tolerance.

Psychological dependence or addiction is not a problem, except in some patients with pre-existing addiction. If alternative methods of pain control are used (such as nerve

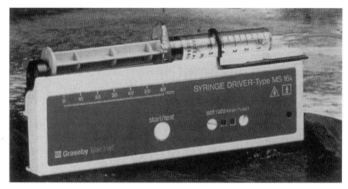

Portable syringe driver for automatic drug infusion

Rationale for alternative opioids

- Basic pharmacology of the drug and particular properties relating to renal, hepatic, and cognitive impairment
- Progress in basic science, which has illuminated the genetic differences between individuals in response to opioids

---

Common adverse effects of opioids

- *Sedation*—Some sedation is common at the start of treatment, but in most patients it resolves within a few days
- *Nausea and vomiting*—Nausea is common in patients taking oral morphine, vomiting rather less so. These are initial side effects and usually resolve over a few days, but they can easily be controlled—metoclopramide (10 mg every eight hours) or haloperidol (1.5 mg at night or twice daily) is effective for most patients
- *Constipation* develops in almost all patients and should be treated prophylactically with laxatives
- *Dry mouth* is often the most troublesome adverse effect for patients. Patients should be advised on simple measures to combat this, such as frequent sips of iced drinks, saliva replacements, or saliva stimulants

blocks) it is usually possible to reduce the dose of the analgesic or even withdraw it without adverse psychological effects. Physical dependence can occur, and this physiological response can manifest itself as a flu-like illness in some patients if an opioid is discontinued suddenly. This can be managed easily by a more gradual withdrawal of the opioid.

Opioid toxicity

There is wide variation, both between individuals and within individuals over time, in the dose of opioid that can be tolerated. Though toxicity can be frightening and life threatening, it is usually reversible if it is diagnosed early.

Opioid toxicity may present as subtle agitation, seeing shadows at the periphery of the visual field, vivid dreams, visual and auditory hallucinations, confusion, and myoclonic jerks. Agitated confusion may be misinterpreted as uncontrolled pain and further opioids given. A vicious cycle then follows, in which the patient is given sedation and may become dehydrated, resulting in the accumulation of opioid metabolites and further toxicity.

Management includes reducing the dose of opioid, ensuring adequate hydration, and treating the agitation with haloperidol (1.5–3 mg orally or subcutaneously, repeated hourly as needed). If toxicity is severe and opioid analgesia is still needed, then a switch in opioid usually leads to a faster recovery. If a different opioid is required, a lower dose than the equianalgesic dose should usually be prescribed.

Before the more sophisticated use of opioids, opioid toxicity was often mislabelled as "terminal agitation."

Opioid responsiveness

Some pains do not respond well to opioids. Although no pain can be assessed as unresponsive to opioids before a careful therapeutic trial of the drug, some pains are more commonly unresponsive. These include bone pain related to movement and some cases of neuropathic pain. Adjuvant drugs, radiotherapy, and anaesthetic block techniques may be helpful in such cases. Radiotherapy provides effective relief of pain from bone metastases in about half of cases—a single fraction is often sufficient, thus avoiding frequent hospital visits. Problems with difficult pain will be addressed in the next chapter.

Factors that affect the ability to tolerate opioids

- The degree of responsiveness of the pain to opioid analgesia
- Previous exposure to opioids
- Rate of titration of the dose
- Concomitant medication
- Concomitant disease
- Genetic factors
- Biochemical factors such as renal function

Further reading

- Doyle D, Hanks G, Cherny NI, Calman K. *Oxford textbook of palliative medicine*. Oxford: Oxford University Press, 2003.
- Sykes N, Fallon M. *Cancer pain*. Arnold: 2002.
- WHO Expert Committee. Cancer pain relief and palliative care. *World Health Organ Tech Rep Ser* 1990;804:1–75.

3 Difficult pain

Lesley Colvin, Karen Forbes, Marie Fallon

Pain occurs in up to 70% of patients with advanced cancer, and in about 65% of patients dying from non-malignant disease. For most of these patients (about 80%) pain can be controlled by using a simple, stepwise approach and a limited number of oral analgesics as set out in the WHO's analgesic ladder (chapter 2). About 10% of patients will require more complex, sometimes invasive, management to control their pain, leaving another 10% with cancer pain that is difficult to control.

This group of patients with "difficult pain" present complex management problems. Their pain often falls into one of three categories: it responds poorly to opioids, it is episodic and breaks through despite background opioid analgesia, or opioids are irrelevant in its management.

Opioid irrelevant pain

Pain is not just a physical experience. Patients with pain that does not respond to escalating doses of opioids should be reassessed and other contributors to their pain explored. "Total pain" is best treated by exploring the underlying issues, rather than using opioids. The term "total pain" is used to describe the final sensation of pain perceived by a patient, acknowledging that this perception can be exaggerated by factors other than a physically noxious stimulus—for example, psychosocial distress.

Pain that responds poorly to opioids

The European Association for Palliative Care (EAPC) guidelines on the use of morphine and alternative opioids in cancer pain confirm oral morphine as the opioid of choice for moderate to severe pain. Dose titration with normal release morphine every four hours, with the same dose for breakthrough pain as required, is suggested. The patient's 24 hour morphine requirement can then be reassessed daily and their regular dose adjusted accordingly. Measures to treat such patients include exploring psychosocial issues, managing the side effects, reducing the dose of opioid, switching to an alternative opioid, or changing the route of administration. The use of adjuvant drugs or co-analgesics may be appropriate, depending on the cause of the pain. Many such patients will have neuropathic pain.

Neuropathic pain

Nociceptive pain results from real or potential tissue damage. Neuropathic pain is caused by damage to the peripheral or central nervous system. A simple definition is "pain in an area of abnormal sensation." Pain may be described as aching, burning, shooting, or stabbing and may be associated with abnormal sensation; normal touch is perceived as painful (allodynia). It may be caused by tumour invasion or compression but also by surgery, radiotherapy, and chemotherapy. Many patients have neuropathic pain that responds to opioids, and so initial management should include a trial of opioids. Patients who remain in pain will require additional measures.

The early addition of adjuvant analgesics, such as a tricyclic antidepressant or an anticonvulsant, should be considered. The number needed to treat is 3 for both categories. There is no evidence for a specific adjuvant for specific descriptors of neuropathic pain.

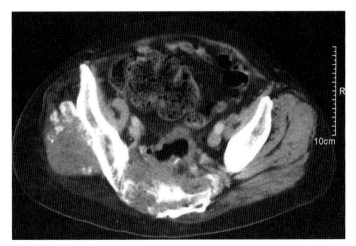

Computed tomography scan showing advanced pelvic disease from colorectal tumour resulting in severe pain

> Patients may be overwhelmed by their situation and the central nervous system can express this as physical pain, though social, psychological, or spiritual factors may be major components

> About 10% of patients will have pain that responds poorly to opioids and is uncontrolled even with a dose of morphine sufficient to give them intolerable side effects

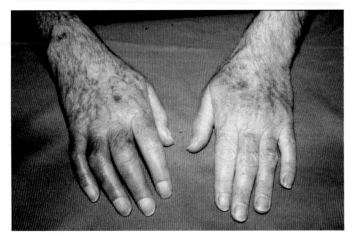

Classical changes associated with a brachial plexopathy due to a right Pancoast tumour: oedema, trophic changes, muscle wasting

In addition, there is no evidence for combining adjuvants. In clinical practice, an adjuvant is chosen for an individual patient after all symptoms and potential side effects are considered. Doses should be titrated to balance analgesia with adverse effects. If titration has reached a limit and pain has only partially responded then a second adjuvant may be added in some cases. This usually means a reduction in the dose of the first. A common example of combining adjuvants is gabapentin, which at maximum tolerated dose can sometimes be reduced to allow the addition of amitriptyline.

Adjuvant analgesics*

Drug	Dose	Indications	Side effects
NSAIDs—for example, diclofenac or COX 2 NSAID (evidence of GI side effects)	50 mg oral every 8 hours (slow release 75 mg every 12 hours); 100 mg per rectum once a day	Bone metastases, soft tissue infiltration, liver pain, inflammatory pain	Gastric irritation and bleeding, fluid retention, headache; caution in renal impairment
Steroids—for example, dexamethasone	8–16 mg a day; use in morning; titrate down to lowest dose that controls pain	Raised intracranial pressure, nerve compression, soft tissue infiltration, liver pain	Gastric irritation if used together with NSAID, fluid retention, confusion, Cushingoid appearance, candidiasis, hyperglycaemia
Gabapentin	100–300 mg nightly (starting dose) (titrate to 600 mg every 8 hours; higher dose may be needed)	Nerve pain of any cause	Mild sedation, tremor, confusion
Amitriptyline (evidence for all tricyclics)	25 mg nightly (starting dose) 10 mg nightly (in elderly patients)	Nerve pain of any cause	Sedation, dizziness, confusion, dry mouth, constipation, urinary retention; avoid in patients with cardiac disease
Carbamazepine (evidence for all anticonvulsants)	100–200 mg nightly (starting dose)	Nerve pain of any cause	Vertigo, sedation, constipation, rash

*Drugs with a primary indication other than pain, but analgesic when used as above.

Non-pharmacological techniques
There are several non-pharmacological techniques for the management of neuropathic pain.

Psychological techniques
Psychological techniques, such as cognitive behavioural therapies, include simple relaxation, hypnosis, and biofeedback. These methods focus on overt behaviour and underlying cognitions and train the patient in coping strategies and behavioural techniques. Though this is clearly of more use in chronic non-malignant pain rather than in patients with cancer pain, simple relaxation techniques should not be forgotten.

Stimulation therapies
Acupuncture has been used successfully in eastern medicine for centuries. There does seem to be a scientific basis for acupuncture, with release of endogenous analgesics within the spinal cord. Acupuncture is particularly useful for myofascial pain, which is a common secondary phenomenon in many cancer pain syndromes.

Transcutaneous electrical nerve stimulation (TENS) may have a similar mechanism of action to acupuncture. There is evidence to support its use in both acute and chronic pain.

Herbal medicine and homoeopathy are widely used for pain, but often with little evidence for efficacy. Regulations on safety for these treatments are limited compared with those for conventional drugs, and doctors should be wary of unrecognised side effects that may result.

TENS for control of neuropathic pain that responds poorly to opioids

Episodic pain

In 2002 an EAPC working group suggested the term episodic pain to describe "any acute transient pain that is severe and has an intensity that flares over baseline." Episodic pain thus encompasses breakthrough pain and incident pain.

Breakthrough pain includes pain returning before the next dose of opioid is due or acute exacerbations of pain occurring on the background of pain usually controlled by an opioid regimen. Incident pain is usually defined as that occurring due to a voluntary action, such as movement or passing urine or stool. Pain due to bony metastases exacerbated by movement or weight bearing can be particularly problematic.

Incident pain

Patients with bony metastases in the spine, pelvis, or femora may have pain that escalates on movement, walking, standing, or even sitting. Opioid analgesics along with non-steroidal anti-inflammatory drugs are the mainstay of treatment, with the aim of making the patient comfortable at rest. Increasing the opioid dose further is often unhelpful as a dose sufficient to make movement possible is too sedating when the resting patient's opioid requirement is decreased. Rescue or breakthrough doses of normal release opioid are usually used in anticipation of movement, along with non-drug measures such as radiotherapy, possible surgery, and appropriate aids and appliances.

Bisphosphonates are interesting drugs established in the prevention of skeletal events due to metastases in most solid tumours. In some patients, analgesia can be achieved acutely, and trial evidence is emerging for good analgesia in pain due to bone metastases.

Interventional techniques

Before interventional techniques are considered, it is important to exclude untreated depression, general anxiety, and distress (though untreated pain may also lead to any or all of these).

Chapter 2 discusses the role of trying a different opioid. The fundamental limiting factor in most patients with uncontrolled difficult pain is the inability to give higher doses because of side effects. It is worthwhile remembering all the strategies to "open the therapeutic window," including using a different drug.

Methadone deserves a special mention in this context. It has unusual properties, which we do not fully understand. It has a different receptor binding profile from the pure μ agonists and can be remarkably potent at small doses.

It is not unusual to achieve markedly superior analgesia and a better side-effect profile with a switch to methadone. In addition, difficult elements of a pain—such as neuropathic or incident pain, or both—may become easier to control.

Starting or switching to methadone can be complicated in some patients, and specialist advice should usually be sought.

Invasive analgesic techniques

Despite appropriate use of analgesia and non-drug therapies, chemotherapy, and radiotherapy by multidisciplinary teams, a considerable number of patients will still have uncontrolled pain or unacceptable side effects, or both.

Such patients should be considered for some form of invasive analgesic technique as part of their overall management. This may range from a simple nerve block to more invasive techniques such as regional or neurodestructive blocks.

The choice of technique is influenced by:

- *Patient's expectations*—Adequate assessment of pain is the first step in management. Involvement of patients and relatives is important and aids decisions about treatment
- *Prognosis and required duration of analgesia*—Although often difficult to predict, prognosis will affect how appropriate any

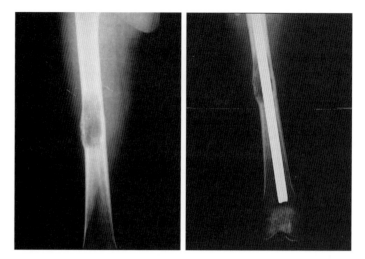

Radiographs showing lystic lesions in femur (left) and internal stabilisation of bone (right)

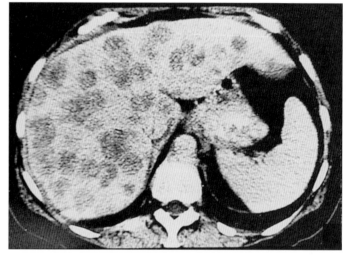

Computed tomogram of enlarged liver due to metastatic spread of cancer (reproduced with permission from Times Mirror International Publishing)

Methadone equianalgesic conversion—seek specialist advice

NB: the ratio depends on the dose of previous opioid
- If morphine 30–90 mg (oral) use ratio of 4:1 (for instance, morphine 30 mg is approximately equivalent to 7 mg of methadone)
- If morphine 90–300 mg (oral) use ratio of 8:1 (for instance, morphine 300 mg (oral) is approximately equivalent to 35 mg methadone (oral))
- If morphine >300 mg (oral) use ratio of 12:1 (for instance, morphine 400 mg (oral) is approximately equivalent to 35 mg methadone (oral))
- If previous morphine dose is *much* higher than 300 mg, the dose ratio will be higher than 12:1

---

particular intervention may be. Further planned oncological treatment may require short term use of interventions for pain control

- *Pathology*—The site and extent of disease will affect the response to analgesics and direct which interventions have a high chance of improving pain control. Plexus or nerve root involvement is common, as is incident pain
- *Personnel*—Early involvement of pain specialists in a multidisciplinary setting is important for planning analgesic strategies. This can help to minimise the length of stay in hospital and reduce problems with severe uncontrolled pain. Local availability of expertise and adequate training of staff and relatives must be considered when technique is selected.

A basic rule is that the technique with the least likelihood of severe side effects should be chosen by using simple techniques before progression to more complex strategies.

In general, neurodestructive techniques should be reserved for when other measures have failed or when life span is obviously limited.

Spinal routes of drug delivery

With improvements in catheter and pump technology, use of spinal lines is becoming more common in pain control. If the technique is carried out by appropriately trained personnel, complication rates are low, allowing flexible, long term analgesia that can be used in an outpatient setting. Catheters can be inserted either into the epidural space or into the subarachnoid (intrathecal) space, where the cerebrospinal fluid is found. The line may be tunnelled subcutaneously to reduce risks of infection and movement of the catheter. The choice of technique depends on several factors.

Drugs

As the patients who need this technique tend to have complex pain problems, multimodal analgesia has the best results. A combination of low dose local anaesthetic, opioid, and clonidine is effective for most patients. Midazolam can be useful as an additional agent, particularly if there are problems with opioid tolerance. If ketamine is used then it should be preservative-free to reduce problems with neurotoxicity. The initial conversion of opioid dose from oral or systemic opioid is variable and depends on the opioid used and comorbidity of the individual patient. Long acting opioids should be stopped before the line is inserted and the patient converted to short acting agents. An approximate dose calculation from subcutaneous diamorphine is:

- Epidural: 1/10 of systemic dose
- Intrathecal: 1/10 of epidural dose

Thus, if a patient was on 100 mg of subcutaneous diamorphine a day, the equivalent epidural dose would be 10 mg and the equivalent intrathecal dose would be 1 mg per 24 hours.

The initial solution used for epidural infusion is normally:

- 9 ml 0.5% bupivacaine
- 75–150 µg clonidine
- Diamorphine according to individual patient.

This gives a total volume of 10 ml infused over 24 hours.

Should there be a major problem with pump malfunction, and the whole syringe were accidentally given at once, this should not give a major life threatening overdose. Education and training of staff is important to minimise potential complications.

The future

Agents not currently widely available in the UK that may be helpful in managing patients with cancer pain include:

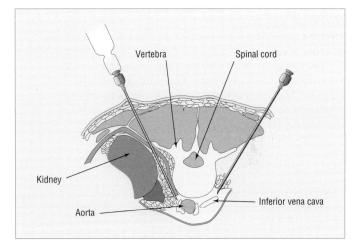

Coeliac plexus nerve block

- *Lidocaine patches*—These are currently available in the US but not in the UK. They have a good side effect profile and studies have shown efficacy in neuropathic pain. We have also used them in our centre for bone pain, particularly vertebral metastases, with some success.
- *Pregabalin*—This agent is a 3-alkylated analogue of GABA (γ-amino butyric acid), with a similar pharmacological profile to gabapentin, acting via the α2/δ subunit on voltage gated calcium channels in the central nervous system. However, it has greater potency than gabapentin. Randomised controlled trials to date have shown efficacy against some forms of neuropathic pain and an improved sleep pattern. Side effects seem similar to those seen with gabapentin. Titration of dose is easier than with gabapentin.
- *N-methyl-d-aspartate (NMDA) subtype selective agents*—Currently available agents are non-selective. There is evidence from animal models that particular subtypes of the NMDA receptor may have potential for analgesia with reduced side effects and opioid sparing effects. These include agents acting at the glycine-B modulatory site or the NR2B subunit.
- *Calcitonin gene-related peptide (CGRP) antagonists*—CGRP is found in sensory neurones. Non-peptide analogues with a favourable pharmacokinetic profile may have potential as analgesics.

Further reading

- Hanks GW, Conno F, Cherny N, Hanna M, Kalso E, Mc Quay HJ, et al. Morphine and alternative opioids in cancer pain: the EAPC recommendations. *Br J Cancer* 2001;84:587–93.
- Mercadante S, Radbruch L, Caraceni A, Cherny N, Kaasa S, Nauck F, et al. Steering Committee of the European Association for Palliative Care (EAPC) Research Network. Episodic (breakthrough) pain: consensus conference of an expert working group of the European Association for Palliative Care. *Cancer* 2002;94:832–9.
- Portenoy R, Forbes K, Lussier D, Hanks GW. Difficult pain problems: an integrated approach. In: Doyle D, Hanks GW, Cherny N, Calman K, eds. *Oxford textbook of palliative medicine.* 3rd ed. Oxford: Oxford University Press, 2003:438–58.
- World Health Organization. *Cancer pain relief.* Geneva: WHO, 1996.
- Zech DF, Grond S, Lynch J, Hertel D, Lehmann KA. Validation of World Health Organization Guidelines for cancer pain relief: a 10-year prospective study. *Pain* 1995;63:65–76.

Potential complications of spinal line

Complication	Sign/symptom	Action
CSF leak	Severe headache (postural)	Lie flat, encourage fluid intake (iv if necessary); blood patch
Infection	Local signs, pyrexia	Avoid—aseptic technique for any dressing changes, line changes etc; antibiotics
Cord compression—may be secondary to tumour, haematoma, abscess	Signs of cord compression—sensory level, weakness, may be pain	Rare, may need surgical treatment
Catheter block or fracture	Acute increase in pain, may be leakage of infusion fluid	Replace catheter
Catheter disconnection	Leakage of infusion fluid from disconnection site	Wrap in sterile saline soaked swab immediately Replace syringe, line, and distal filter

Complications related to drugs

Complication	Sign/symptom	Action
Opioid withdrawal	Agitation, insomnia, etc	Increase opioid dose either via catheter or short acting oral dose
Opioid toxicity	Hallucinations, sedation, twitching, respiratory depression	Decrease dose, stop opioids by other routes, use naloxone if clinically important respiratory depression
Acute opioid tolerance	Requiring rapid dose escalation despite stable situation with tumour	Add midazolam to infusion mixture, switch to different opioid
Pruritus—uncommon with long term use	Itching—often nasal	Naloxone (low dose), change or stop opioid
Urinary retention—more common in men	Unable to pass urine	Catheterise
Excess motor block	Leg weakness	Decrease local anaesthetic dose

4 Breathlessness, cough, and other respiratory problems

Carol Davis, Gillian Percy

Respiratory problems are common in patients with advanced incurable disease. This article describes palliation in adults with malignant disease, but the principles can be applied to many types of non-malignant disease.

A detailed history, examination, and appropriate investigations are needed to establish the most likely cause of any symptom. The degree of functional impairment should be assessed, as should the influence of factors that affect the severity of the symptom, including pre-existing diseases (for example, chronic obstructive pulmonary disease, COPD), exacerbating factors (for example, anaemia, ascites, or profound anxiety), and additional factors (for example, pulmonary embolism, infection, or left ventricular failure). All influence management.

Breathlessness

Breathlessness has non-physical as well as physical aspects and, like pain, can be defined by what a patient says it is. It is the unpleasant sensation of being unable to breathe easily. It is common in the terminal stages of cancer: in one survey 70% of 1700 patients experienced breathlessness during their last six weeks of life. It is a particularly distressing and frightening symptom, not only for patients but also for carers. Activity, levels of anxiety, speed of onset, and previous experience may influence patients' perception of breathlessness and its severity.

While there is often an obvious cause (such as pleural effusion or extrinsic bronchial compression), in some patients no cause is found despite thorough assessment. Little is known about the effects of cachexia on respiratory muscle function; hyperventilation may account for breathlessness in some cases.

Management

Management of a breathless patient should be individualised, but some general principles apply. Many members of an interdisciplinary team can contribute. As well as nursing and medical input, physiotherapy is often helpful, particularly for advice on techniques for conserving breathing, positioning, control of panic, and relaxation methods. Occupational therapists can give essential advice on strategies and practical aids for daily activities. There is good evidence to support breathlessness clinics led by nurses.

In selected patients specific treatment, such as anticancer therapy, can improve control of symptoms and quality of life. The appropriateness of various strategies varies with time, but, for many patients, the disadvantages of travelling to a distant or regional centre may be justified when weighed against symptomatic relief gained from radiotherapy, laser therapy, or stenting of an endobronchial tumour. Pleurodesis should be considered early rather than after repeated pleural aspirations as nearly all patients experience recurrence one month after simple aspiration.

Oxygen

Oxygen is usually seen as a non-specific treatment for breathlessness. Patients can become highly dependent on oxygen therapy; many see it as their lifeline. In patients with chronic lung and heart disease, however, there is good evidence that oxygen therapy is beneficial only in specific situations such as hypoxia or pulmonary hypertension.

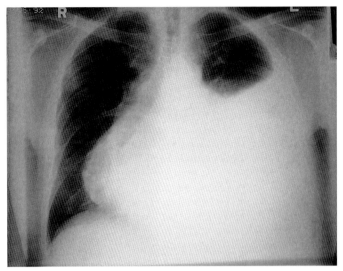

Radiograph of patient with malignant pericardial effusion and secondary pleural effusion causing breathlessness

---

General principles of managing breathlessness

- Reassurance to patient, family, and non-professional and professional carers
- Explanation
- Advice on techniques to conserve breathing, positioning
- Stream of air such as fan or open window
- Distraction and relaxation techniques
- Consider blood transfusion if patient is anaemic
- Encourage adaptations in lifestyle and expectations

Therapeutic options for specific situations

Pleural effusion
- Pleural aspiration with or without pleurodesis
- Pleuroperitoneal shunt

Pericardial effusion
- Aspiration, with or without percutaneous fenestration

Lymphangitis
- High dose corticosteroids

Endobronchial disease
- High dose corticosteroids
- Laser therapy
- Cryotherapy
- Stenting

It is not clear whether oxygen is better than air at relieving breathlessness in patients with advanced cancer; further research is needed to identify which patients are most likely to benefit. Meanwhile, the pros and cons of oxygen therapy should be considered on an individual basis. Not all breathless patients are hypoxaemic and, in any case, not all hypoxaemic patients benefit from oxygen therapy. It seems sensible to prescribe a therapeutic trial of oxygen to patients with resting oxygen saturation concentrations <90%. At the least, some form of objective assessment of the benefits, or not, of oxygen in an individual patient should be performed; and oximetry may be helpful. If relatively long term use is likely, an oxygen concentrator rather than cylinders should be considered for patients at home. The use of nasal speculae can avoid some of the inconvenience of a mask. The gas can be humidified, but this is noisy.

Few patients require continuous oxygen. For others, explanation and individualised coping strategies, including a bedside or hand held fan, sometimes combined with non-specific drug measures, such as opioids or anxiolytics, are more appropriate and often more successful.

Coping with anxiety and panic

The vicious cycle in which anxiety aggravates breathlessness and breathlessness, in turn, creates further anxiety is experienced to some degree by most breathless patients, regardless of the cause. Some may experience a severe panic attack and become convinced that they are about to die. Such attacks are more common than is acknowledged. Patients should be advised of measures that they can initiate to allow them to regain control. These have been summarised as "Stop, purse lips, drop (shoulders), and flop." It is important to teach lay and professional carers how to cope; simple strategies such as gently massaging the breathless person's back can be helpful.

Research on the use of benzodiazepines in breathless patients with chronic non-malignant lung disease is equivocal and, in patients with cancer, does not support their use in unselected patients. If anxiety seems to be a major component or trigger of breathlessness and cannot be relieved by non-pharmacological measures, then a therapeutic trial of a low dose benzodiazepine either regularly or as required seems sensible. Concern about possible respiratory depression is usually unfounded, and any such concern should be weighed against the potential benefit of treatment.

Opioids

The relation between opioids and respiration is not simple; if used inappropriately, opioids can induce respiratory depression, which is determined by pathophysiology, previous exposure to opioids, rate and route of dose titration, and coexisting pathology. However, low dose oral opioids can improve breathlessness, sometimes dramatically, though the precise mechanism of action is unknown.

The dose of opioid can be titrated in the same way as when it is used for pain control, but lower doses and smaller increments should be used. In patients not previously exposed to opioids, as little as 2.5 mg of normal release morphine every four hours may be sufficient. If a patient is already receiving controlled release morphine, many convert to a normal release preparation and allow for a dose increment. For patients unable to swallow, subcutaneous diamorphine can be used. Concurrent laxatives should be prescribed.

Nebulised drugs

If a trial of a nebulised drug is thought appropriate, then nebulised normal saline should be used in the first instance.

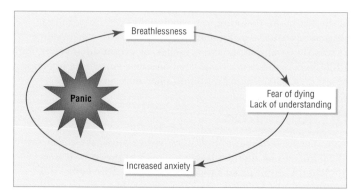

Potential advantages and disadvantages of oxygen treatment

Advantages	Disadvantages
• Reverse hypoxia	• Claustrophobia
• Sense of wellbeing	• Discomfort
• Patients, families, and professionals feel they are doing something	• Drying effect
	• Difficulties in communication
	• Distancing
	• Risk of patient/relatives smoking
	• Cost

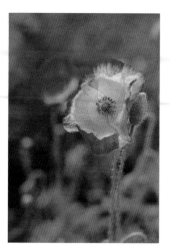

Cycle of increasing panic and breathlessness

Advice to patient about "panic attacks"

• Try to stay calm
• Purse your lips
• Relax shoulders, back, neck, and arms; let your muscles breathe with you, not against you
• Concentrate on breathing out slowly (if breathing in seems difficult)

The opium poppy, *Papaver somniferum* (photos.com)

Inhaled bronchodilators should be reserved for patients with reversible airways obstruction. Trials of nebulised morphine have been conducted in healthy volunteers and in patients with COPD and malignant disease. Current evidence does not support its use. Other nebulised drugs should be regarded as experimental in these patients.

Cough

Cough is a normal but complex physiological mechanism, under both voluntary and involuntary control, that protects the lungs by removing mucus and foreign matter from the larynx, trachea, and bronchi. Pathological cough is common in malignant and non-malignant disease and can be classified in various ways. Several causes may coexist in one patient. Malignant disease may cause mechanical distortion of the airways causing dry cough (for example, by pulmonary effusion or endobronchial tumour) or accumulation of material within the airway causing a cough productive of blood, mucus, or purulent sputum.

Management

Management should be determined by the type and cause of the cough as well as the patient's general condition and likely prognosis. When possible, the main aim should be to reverse or ameliorate the cause, combined with appropriate symptomatic measures. Exacerbating factors should be defined and simple measures, such as a change in posture, particularly at night, can be helpful. Breathlessness can trigger cough, and vice versa. Persistent cough can also precipitate vomiting, exhaustion, chest or abdominal pain, rib fracture, syncope, and insomnia.

Cough suppressants are usually used to manage dry cough, except in irritant nocturnal cough and cough in dying patients. The most effective antitussive agents are the opioids. Opioids such as codeine or pholcodine are mild antitussives; morphine and comparable drugs have a more pronounced effect. Normal release morphine, administered as a tablet or solution, should be tried if regular administration of codeine or pholcodine is ineffective, starting at a dose of 5–10 mg either regularly every four hours or as needed. The dose can be titrated in the same way as for pain relief (see chapter 2). Methadone linctus can be particularly effective at night because it has a long half life, but the risk of accumulation exists.

Mucolytic treatments such as simple linctus or nebulised saline may benefit patients with a wet unproductive cough. Use of nebulised saline can result in the production of copious liquid sputum, and this makes it unsuitable for those who are unable to expectorate.

Nebulised local anaesthetics can relieve intractable, unproductive cough. Bronchospasm can occur, not necessarily only with the first dose, and so nebulised bronchodilators should be available, at least when treatment is initiated. Both lignocaine (up to 5 ml of 2% solution every six hours) and bupivacaine (up to 5 ml of 0.25% solution every eight hours) have been used; relative efficacy and toxicity has not been established. Treatment reduces the sensitivity of the gag reflex and causes a transitory hoarseness. Patients should not eat or drink for an hour after nebulisation.

Antibiotics can be used to treat chest infection and to relieve pain, insomnia, or distress associated with a productive cough. There is anecdotal evidence that a single intravenous or large oral dose of a broad spectrum antibiotic can reduce infected secretions, even in dying patients. The decision on whether to treat an infection with antibiotics may raise ethical dilemmas and needs careful consideration and discussion. Chest physiotherapy should be considered in all patients.

Common causes of cough

Non-malignant

Acute infection
- Upper respiratory viral infection
- Bronchopneumonia

Airway disease
- Asthma
- COPD

Irritant
- Foreign body
- Cigarette smoke
- Oesophageal reflux

Cardiovascular causes
- Left ventricular failure

Chronic infection
- Cystic fibrosis
- Bronchiectasis
- Postnasal drip

Recurrent aspiration
- Motor neurone disease
- Multiple sclerosis

Drug induced
- Angiotensin converting enzyme inhibitors
- Inhaled drugs

Parenchymal disease
- Interstitial fibroses

Malignant

Airway obstruction
- Endobronchial disease

Pleural disease
- Pleural effusion
- Mesothelioma

Vocal cord palsy
- Hilar tumour or lymphadenopathy

Interstitial disease
- Lymphangitis
- Multiple pulmonary metastases
- Radiation pneumonia

Classification of types of cough

- Productive cough, patient able to cough effectively
- Productive cough, patient not able to cough effectively
- Non-productive cough

Pharmacological agents that inhibit cough

Opioids and opioid derivatives
- Codeine phosphate
- Dextromethorphan
- Pholcodine
- Methadone
- Morphine

Corticosteroids
- Prednisolone
- Dexamethasone
(Often used to relieve cough related to endobronchial tumour, lymphangitis, or radiation pneumonia)

Local anaesthetics

Lozenges
- Benzocaine
- Lignocaine
(For laryngeal, pharyngeal, or tracheal irritation)

Bronchodilators

- Salbutamol
- Ipratropium
(Can relieve cough associated with reversible airways obstruction)

Nebulised
- Lignocaine
- Bupivacaine
(Useful for intractable, unproductive cough, use with care)

Therapeutic options in managing productive cough

Tenacious sputum
- Steam inhalation
- Nebulised saline
- Simple linctus
- Physiotherapy
- Active cycle breathing

Heart failure
- Diuretics

Purulent sputum
- Antibiotics
- Postural drainage
- Physiotherapy
- Cough suppression

Loose secretions but unable to cough
- Positioning
- Anti-muscarinic drugs
- Suction

Antimuscarinics—In some patients it is more appropriate to reduce salivary secretion. Hyoscine hydrobromide or glycopyrronium bromide can be given as a subcutaneous injection or by subcutaneous infusion over 24 hours (see chapter 11).

Haemoptysis

In many studies of patients with haemoptysis, a definitive cause is established in only half. Even in patients with a proved malignancy, haemoptysis can be due to other causes. While lung cancer is the commonest cause of massive haemoptysis (>200 ml/24 hours), non-malignant disorders such as acute bronchitis, bronchiectasis, and pulmonary embolism can cause mild to moderate haemoptysis.

Management

It is important to establish that the blood or blood stained material has come from the lungs or bronchial tubes and not the nose, upper respiratory tract, or gastrointestinal tract. Management depends on the volume of blood lost, the cause, and prognosis. Radiotherapy (endobronchial or external beam) and laser therapy are effective in controlling bleeding from an endobronchial tumour in over three quarters of patients.

Massive haemoptysis should be regarded as an emergency, whether or not resuscitation is appropriate. Patients bleeding as a result of a non-malignant cause may warrant active management, but this is rarely the case in those with advanced lung malignancy. Palliative management should be aimed at reducing awareness and fear. A combination of parenterally administered strong opioid and a benzodiazepine is usually required. The intravenous route should be used if there is peripheral vascular shutdown. The patient's family and staff will need support during and after a death from massive haemoptysis. It is often possible to predict the likelihood of a massive bleed and plan for such a crisis in several ways, including establishing an emergency supply of appropriate drugs in the patient's home.

Stridor

A harsh inspiratory wheezing sound results from obstruction of the larynx or major airways. Treatment with corticosteroids (such as dexamethasone 16 mg daily) can provide rapid relief. Explanation should always be given, together with advice about sitting or lying as upright as possible and measures to relieve anxiety. Inhalation of a mixture of helium and oxygen (in a ratio 4:1) is often helpful. Radiotherapy or endoscopic insertion of a tracheal or bronchial stent should be considered but are not always appropriate.

Pleural and chest wall pain

Pleural and chest wall pain may exacerbate breathlessness and may be difficult to manage. Non-pharmacological measures such as TENS or acupuncture may be helpful. Analgesics should be prescribed in a stepwise fashion (see chapter 2). Cough suppression may help. Radiotherapy should be considered if the pain is caused by metastases in the bones or soft tissues. An intercostal nerve block may temporarily alleviate pain from rib metastases or fracture. Percutaneous cordotomy can be effective for the relief of chest wall pain such as that commonly caused by mesothelioma (see chapter 3, Difficult pain).

Therapeutic options for haemoptysis	
Minor bleed	**Major bleed**
Caused by lung tumour	*Resuscitation appropriate*
● Oral haemostatic drug—such as tranexamic acid	● Establish intravenous access
● Radiotherapy—external beam or endobronchial	● Transfusion
● Laser therapy	● Bronchoscopy and endoscopic measures
	● Bronchial artery embolisation
	● Open surgery
Caused by pulmonary embolism	*Resuscitation inappropriate*
● Anticoagulation	● Intravenous opioid and benzodiazepine
Any cause	
● Treat coagulation disorder if present	
● Cough suppressant	
Both situations	
● Patient should be nursed lying on his or her side, on the side of the tumour	
● Mask evidence of bleed—such as with red or green towels	
● Calm witnesses—patient, family, staff, other patients	

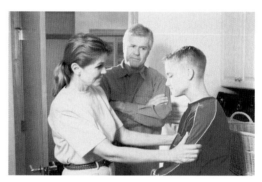

Families need support after a death from massive haemoptysis (photos.com)

Careful judgement is required in deciding whether to discuss the risk of massive haemoptysis with a patient and relatives

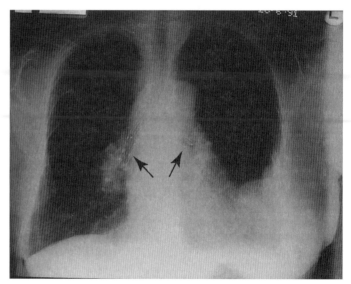

Radiograph showing bilateral bronchial stents in patient with obstructive lesion

5 Oral health in patients with advanced disease

Jeremy Bagg, Andrew Davies

Oral problems are common among patients in palliative care, particularly those with advanced cancer. The aetiology of oral problems includes a direct effect of underlying disease; an indirect effect of underlying disease; an effect of treatment for underlying disease; an effect of a concomitant disease or treatment for concomitant disease; or a combination of all of these.

Oral problems are an important cause of physical, psychological, and social morbidity among these patients.

Straightforward oral hygiene can prevent many problems, and relatively simple interventions can often resolve them. Successful management, however, depends on adequate assessment—that is, providing "the right treatment for the right disease."

Patients seldom report oral symptoms or problems. Thus, healthcare professionals should always ask patients about oral symptoms, and examine them for oral signs. Indeed, an oral assessment is a mandatory part of the overall assessment of these patients. Such an assessment needs to be repeated on a regular basis as changes may occur within a relatively short period of time.

Prevalence of oral problems in studies involving palliative care patients with cancer

Problem	Prevalence (%)
Oral symptoms	
Dry mouth	58–78
Oral discomfort	33–55
Taste disturbance	26–44
Difficulty chewing	23–52
Difficulty swallowing	23–37
Difficulty speaking	31–59
Halitosis	48
Oral infections	
Oral candidosis	8–83
Dental caries	20–35
Periodontal disease	36

Oral hygiene

The importance of providing regular oral care cannot be overstated. Oral hygiene measures should be performed at least twice a day, if they are to benefit the patient.

The single most important measure is brushing the teeth. A small headed brush, with medium texture nylon filament bristles, is recommended. Soft toothbrushes can be used for patients whose mouths are particularly sore. Patients should be encouraged to use toothpaste containing at least 1000 ppm fluoride. For patients who have difficulty rinsing their mouths or swallowing and are at increased risk of aspiration, a non-foaming alternative such as chlorhexidine gluconate gel should be used. Water alone is acceptable for those who cannot tolerate toothpaste.

For very debilitated patients, chemical plaque control may be helpful. The most effective antiplaque agent is chlorhexidine, which should be used no more than twice daily. Chlorhexidine will not remove established plaque so the mouth should be thoroughly cleaned, ideally by a dentist or dental hygienist, before regular use of chlorhexidine to maintain a plaque-free environment. Chlorhexidine is used most commonly as a 0.2% mouthwash (10 ml twice a day) but is also available as a 1% gel and a 0.2% spray.

Denture hygiene

Dentures are readily colonised by microorganisms so it is essential that a high level of denture hygiene is maintained. Denture care must be carried out at least once a day, preferably at night. All dentures, both partial and complete, must be cleaned outside the mouth and the soft tissues of the mouth and standing teeth cleaned separately. Dentures should always be cleaned over a bowl of water, so that if dropped they will not be damaged. Commercial products are available for cleaning dentures, but household soap, or just water alone, is satisfactory. Ordinary toothpaste should not be used because it is too abrasive. The denture should be rinsed well before re-insertion.

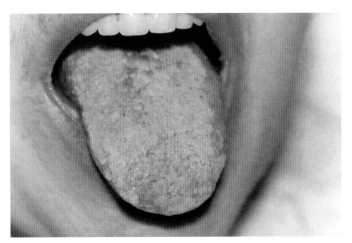

This patient had a drug induced dry mouth, which resulted in poor oral hygiene, halitosis, and oral candidosis: the oral symptoms led to low mood, while the halitosis led to limited physical contact between the patient and her family

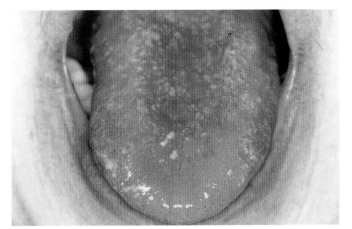

The same patient as above. Her mouth dramatically improved when she was treated with a saliva stimulant

Dentures should be left out of the mouth at night. Plastic dentures should be soaked overnight in a dilute solution of sodium hypochlorite (such one part 1% Milton to 80 parts water). This allows disinfection of the denture and reduces the likelihood of denture stomatitis (see below). The denture should be rinsed well under running water before being returned to the patient's mouth. Dentures with metal parts should be soaked in chlorhexidine gluconate (0.2% solution) to achieve disinfection. Dentures should be stored in a denture container clearly marked with the patient's name. Dentures themselves can also be marked with the patient's name.

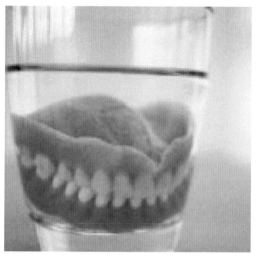

Dentures in Milton

Oral symptoms

Dry mouth (xerostomia)

Xerostomia may be caused by a reduction in the secretion of saliva, a change in the composition of saliva, or a combination of these factors.

Xerostomia is associated with several other oral symptoms and problems, including oral discomfort, disturbance in taste, difficulty chewing, difficulty swallowing, difficulty speaking, difficulty in retaining dentures, dental caries, oral candidosis, and other oral infections. The various manifestations of xerostomia reflect the multiple functions of saliva.

The management of xerostomia involves treatment of the underlying cause and use of saliva stimulants or use of saliva substitutes. The choice of symptomatic treatment will depend on several factors, including the aetiology of the xerostomia, the patient's general condition, the presence or absence of teeth, and, most importantly, the patient's preference.

There are good theoretical reasons for prescribing saliva stimulants rather than saliva substitutes. Furthermore, in the studies that have compared both, patients have generally preferred the saliva stimulants. The management of dry mouth also involves oral hygiene measures and the use of fluoride supplements.

Acidic products are relatively contraindicated in dentate patients and should be used with caution in edentulous patients. A low pH predisposes to dental erosion, dental caries, and oral candidosis. It should be noted that some of the artificial salivas are acidic in nature.

Oral discomfort and pain

A dry mouth, poorly fitting dentures, intraoral diseases (malignant, infectious), local radiotherapy, and systemic chemotherapy can all cause oral discomfort in patients in palliative care. The strategies used to manage oral discomfort include treatment of the underlying cause, topical analgesics (local anaesthetics, other agents), and systemic agents.

Taste disturbance

Similarly, there are several potential causes of taste disturbance, including dry mouth, intraoral diseases (malignant, infectious), local surgery, local radiotherapy, systemic chemotherapy, drug treatment, and zinc deficiency.

Halitosis

Halitosis may be "physiological" (no underlying disease present) or "pathological" (underlying disease present). Physiological halitosis results from the bacterial putrefaction of food, epithelial cells, blood cells, and saliva; the process occurs mainly on the dorsal surface of the tongue. This is the most common type of halitosis. Pathological halitosis usually results from disease of the oral cavity but may also be associated with disease of the respiratory or gastrointestinal tract or a systemic metabolic problem. There are several strategies for the

---

Some causes of dry mouth

- Drug treatment (most common cause)
  Many drugs used in palliative care (for example, analgesics and antiemetics)
- Local tumour
- Local surgery
- Local radiotherapy
- Dehydration

Management of dry mouth

Treat the underlying cause

Saliva substitutes
- Water
- Artificial saliva—for example, mucin based, CMC* based
- Other agents

Saliva stimulants
- Chewing gum
- Organic acids—for example, malic acid, citric acid
- Parasympathomimetic drugs—for example, pilocarpine hydrochloride, bethanechol chloride
- Other agents
- Acupuncture

*Carboxymethylcellulose

Management of taste disturbance

Treat the underlying cause

Dietary interventions
- Use foods that taste "good"
- Avoid foods that taste "bad"
- Enhance the taste of the food (use salt, sugar, and other flavourings)
- Focus on the presentation, smell, consistency, and temperature of the food

Zinc supplements

management of physiological halitosis; the management of pathological halitosis involves treatment of the underlying disease.

Management strategies for physiological halitosis

Mechanical measures to reduce bacterial numbers/nutrients
- Teeth cleaning
- Use of interdental aids (dental floss, dental sticks)
- Tongue cleaning (toothbrush, tongue scraper)
- Periodontal treatment (scaling, root planing)

Chemical measures to reduce bacterial numbers/nutrients
- Chlorhexidine (in mouthwash)
- Other antimicrobial agents—for example, baking soda, cetylperidinium, essential oils, hydrogen peroxide, triclosan (in various vehicles*)

Chemical measures to counteract odour
- Zinc salts (in mouthwashes, toothpastes, or chewing gum)
- Other agents—for example, baking soda, chlorine dioxide (in various vehicles*)

Dietary modification

Smoking cessation

Masking agents
- For example, mints, cosmetic sprays/mouthwashes

Natural products
For example, black tea, various herbs

*Mouthwashes, toothpastes, chewing gum

Oral infections

Fungal infections (oral candidosis)

Oral candidosis is the most common oral infection in palliative care. The predisposing factors include dry mouth, dentures, and immunosuppression. *Candida albicans* is responsible for most oral fungal infections, but other species such as *C glabrata*, *C dubliniensis*, and *C tropicalis* are also important.

Oral candidosis may present in several different clinical forms, including pseudomembranous, erythematous, denture stomatitis, and angular cheilitis. Oral candidosis may spread locally to cause oesophageal candidosis or more widely to cause systemic candidosis.

The management of oral candidosis involves treatment of any predisposing factors (such as disinfection of dentures), together with treatment of the infection with topical or systemic antifungal drugs. Topical treatments for oral candidosis include nystatin, amphotericin B, and miconazole. Topical treatments can be effective, although this depends on correct use. Many palliative care patients find it difficult to comply with the recommended treatment regimens.

Systemic treatments for oral candidosis include fluconazole, itraconazole, and ketoconazole. Systemic treatments tend to be effective and are particularly useful in widespread disease. The drawbacks of these drugs are their contraindications, drug interactions, and the emergence of antifungal drug resistance. Resistance to the azole group of drugs seems to be a growing problem in palliative care, though for most patients in this setting they are generally still effective.

Bacterial infections

Dental caries and periodontal disease are both common among patients in palliative care. Established disease requires specific interventions from the dental team. Oral hygiene measures will help to prevent progression of disease (see above). Other bacterial infections are relatively uncommon.

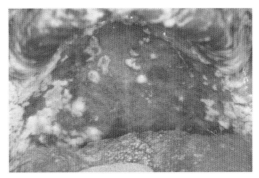

Pseudomembranous candidosis ("oral thrush") (courtesy of Prof David Wray)

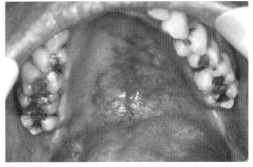

Erythematous candidosis (courtesy of Prof David Wray)

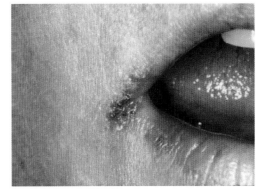

Angular cheilitis (courtesy of Prof David Wray)

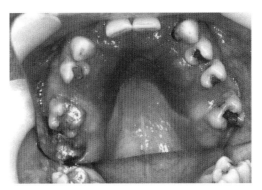

Denture stomatitis (courtesy of Prof David Wray)

Viral infections

Infection with herpes simplex virus (HSV) is relatively common. Most infections are secondary (reactivation) infections. Patients may develop the classic herpes labialis ("cold sore") or, if immunosuppressed, they may develop an atypical picture of oral ulceration/inflammation. The lesions are usually painful, and patients have problems drinking and eating. The treatment involves antiviral treatment (such as aciclovir), together with supportive therapy (such as analgesics).

Dental and denture problems

Involvement of the dental surgeon and other members of the dental team is essential to the management of these problems.

Problems with dentures are common in patients with advanced disease. The underlying cause is usually poor fitting, which leads to difficulty in eating or speaking and possibly oral ulceration. The management of denture problems depends on the physical condition of the patient: fit patients can have their dentures replaced with a copying technique, while less fit patients can have their dentures adjusted or relined. The latter technique can be undertaken at home.

Dental problems are less common because of the high levels of denture wearing within the normal population. Many dental techniques can also be undertaken in the home.

Oral problems in patients with advanced non-malignant disease

Oral problems are common in all groups of patients with advanced disease. Many of these problems are generic in nature (see above), but some are more specific to the individual groups of patients. For example, patients with HIV and AIDS may develop various infectious and malignant problems, including hairy leukoplakia, periodontal disease related to HIV, and Kaposi's sarcoma.

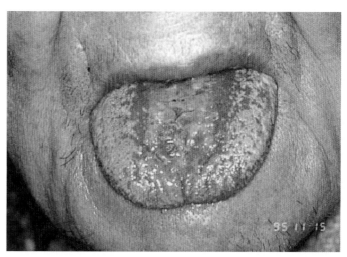

Reactivation of herpes simplex virus infection in immunosuppressed patient (courtesy of Dr Petrina Sweeney)

Further reading

- Davies A, Finlay I. *Oral care in advanced disease*. Oxford: Oxford University Press, 2004.
- Laskaris G. *Colour atlas of oral diseases*. 2nd ed. Stuttgart: Georg Thieme Verlag, 1994.
- Bagg J, MacFarlane TW, Poxton IR, Miller CH, Smith AJ. *Essentials of microbiology for dental students*. Oxford: Oxford University Press, 1999.

6 Anorexia, cachexia, nutrition, and fatigue

Kenneth Fearon, Matthew Barber

What is cachexia?

Cachexia, anorexia, and fatigue are an overlapping and often neglected group of symptoms that at some stage affect most patients with cancer. Similar symptoms may be seen in other conditions, including advanced cardiac failure, COPD, renal failure, and AIDS and in patients who have been in intensive care units. The term cachexia is derived from the Greek words *kakos* and *hexis* meaning poor condition. Cachexia is a broad heterogeneous syndrome. The key feature is wasting that cannot be easily or completely reversed by an increase in food intake alone. Anorexia or reduced appetite often accompanies cachexia. Some patients with anorexia, however, do not have cachexia. Equally some cachectic patients become wasted but apparently do not have anorexia. Fatigue is a common element but again this can occur in isolation.

Cachexia is complex and multifactorial. A patient's evident chronic negative energy and protein balance is most commonly driven by a combination of reduced food intake and metabolic change. Symptoms can include anorexia, early satiety, taste changes, loss of physical function, and fatigue. Signs may include muscle wasting, loss of subcutaneous fat, and peripheral oedema. Different symptoms may predominate in individual patients and may also change with time. Advanced cachexia is generally easy to recognise, but the early symptoms may be more subtle. An unintentional loss of weight of more than 10% with an appropriate underlying diagnosis has traditionally been used as a definition of cachexia. This definition, however, neglects other relevant symptoms and if used rigidly is likely to delay diagnosis and therefore treatment. Equally, with an ever increasing tendency towards obesity in the general population, lesser degrees of weight loss are likely to identify a proportion of patients who, while at risk of developing cachexia, may still be above ideal body weight.

Why is cachexia important?

Anorexia and fatigue are consistently among the most common symptoms reported by patients with advanced cancer. Cachexia affects over 80% of such patients or patients with AIDS before death. It is particularly common in those with solid tumours of the upper gastrointestinal tract and lung. Those with cachexia have reduced survival, often experience anorexia and fatigue, have an altered body image, and have impaired physical activity and overall quality of life. Response to antineoplastic therapy is reduced and morbidity caused by treatment increased. Cachexia is usually progressive and is sometimes fatal.

Does this patient have cachexia?

A history and physical examination are probably the most useful tools in making the diagnosis and assessing response to therapy. Weight loss in the past six months should be recorded. Symptoms associated with reduced food intake (for example, loss of appetite, early satiety, nausea or vomiting, and alterations in taste or smell) are key warning signals. Weight should be measured and recorded along with height. Oedema and ascites are common and should be documented because fluid retention may mask the severity of underlying weight loss. Body mass index (weight (kg)/height (m)^2) should be calculated. A BMI <18 indicates severe undernutrition. The plasma albumin

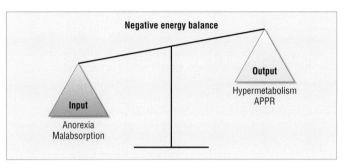

Cachexia is multifactorial, and it effects a patient's balance of negative energy (APPR = acute phase protein response)

The progression through cachexia

Diagnosis of cachexia

Early
- 5% weight loss

Late
- >15% weight loss (BMI 18; albumin <30 g/l)

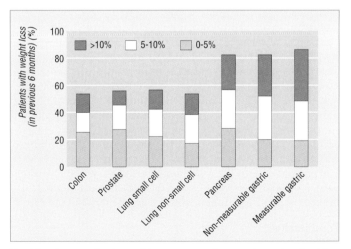

Nutritional status of patients with cancer: prevalence and severity of weight loss

concentration may be low and, if it is accompanied by a raised C reactive protein (CRP) or erythrocyte sedimentation rate (ESR), probably reflects an underlying systemic inflammatory response that may contribute to the weight loss.

Why do patients become cachectic?

The cachectic patient is like an accelerating car running out of petrol. Anorexia critically reduces fuel supply (by about 300–500 kcal (1254–2090 kJ) a day), while accelerated metabolic cycling (for example, glucose-lactate cycling) drives hypermetabolism (100–200 kcal a day). In addition, there are direct catabolic effects at the level of skeletal muscle (for example, activation of the ubiquitin-proteasome pathway) and adipose tissue. The mediators of these changes are complex and include proinflammatory cytokines, stress hormones, and tumour specific cachectic factors such as proteolysis inducing factor (PIF). The main energy (subcutaneous fat) and labile protein reserves (skeletal muscle) of the body are mobilised and the patient becomes prone to secondary effects such as insulin resistance and further muscle wasting due to immobility. These changes underlie a key paradox of cachexia in that while the metabolic rate may be increased, overall (or total) energy expenditure is decreased due to a fall in physical activity.

Management

Once a patient has become severely wasted and bed bound and is within weeks of dying it is unlikely that intervention can have any objective benefit. The longstanding practice of giving such patients steroids to improve mood and perhaps appetite remains a keystone of clinical practice.

At the other extreme of intervention is the patient with incurable cancer, who has a prognosis measured in months, but who has malnutrition related to gut failure because of localised and relatively stable intra-abdominal malignancy. A proportion of these patients benefit from total parenteral nutrition at home. Although not often used in the UK, such intervention, if guided by expert clinical judgment, can result in improved quality and quantity of life. Other groups who may benefit from artificial nutritional support but via the enteral route include patients with slowly advancing head and neck tumours.

Therapeutic principles of management

For most patients the management of cachexia requires insight and enthusiasm from the physician, surgeon, general practitioner, nurse specialist, and dietician with whom the patient may come into contact. Cachexia is a chronic problem for which there is no quick fix and which requires repeated re-evaluation as the clinical condition of the patient changes. Once signs of cachexia are evident patients generally have two to six months to live. Early recognition and prophylactic measures are better than trying to reverse an advanced situation. Good clinical judgment is paramount to identify all reversible factors that may be contributing to the patient's wasting syndrome. In particular, if nausea and vomiting can be controlled with regular antiemetics (or surgery if there is a defined mechanical obstruction), malabsorption treated with enzyme supplements, constipation treated with laxatives, pain well controlled with the minimum of sedation, and depression treated with antidepressants then this sets the background for optimal appetite and function of the gastrointestinal tract.

Food intake

With the recognition that weight loss in patients with cancer is most commonly due to a combination of reduced food intake

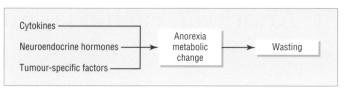

Mediators of cachexia

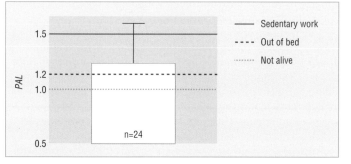

Physical activity level (PAL) in patients with cachexia (adapted from Moses et al, *Br J Cancer* 2004;90:996–1002)

Focus of treatment in cachexia

- Multidisciplinary
- Start early rather than late
- Target reduced food intake and metabolic stress
- Aim to improve physical activity/quality of life
- Nutritional status is not an end in itself

Therapeutic principles

- Exclude/treat obstruction, infections, malabsorption, drug related problems
- Optimise pain control, encourage exercise
- Optimise nutritional intake—varied, attractive food offered at appropriate times in appropriate quantities
- Consider specific anticachectic therapy

---

and metabolic change, once the overall management of the cachectic patient has been optimised, therapeutic strategies should try to address both these issues.

Intake of food can be improved by providing small and frequent meals that are dense in energy and easy to eat (for example, dairy products, ice cream). Patients should eat in pleasant surroundings, and attention should be given to the presentation of food. If, however, patients are unable to finish meals, relatives should be counselled to avoid conflict over the issue. Formal dietary assessment and advice may be sought from a dietician. Provision of energy and protein dense oral sip feeds (1.5 kcal/ml) can often be useful. Care has to be taken that these do not replace normal food. Asking the patient to take a fixed dose at regular times (as with a prescription medication) is one way of optimising compliance. Patients should aim to take 200–400 ml daily (that is, 300–600 kcal), accepting that this will suppress some normal food intake but provide a net gain of 200–400 kcal a day.

When a patient complains of severe anorexia or early satiety it may be necessary to provide an appetite stimulant. Moderate alcohol consumption before and during a meal may help. Prednisolone (5 mg three times a day) or dexamethasone (4 mg a day) can improve appetite and mood but are not generally suitable for long term use (that is, more than six to eight weeks) due to loss of efficacy and side effects including muscle wasting. Progestogens (for example, megestrol acetate 480 mg a day or medroxyprogesterone acetate 1000 mg a day) can improve appetite in about 70% of patients and can also result in increased food intake and weight gain in a smaller proportion (about 20%) of patients. Such effects may in part be due to corticosteroid-like activity: improved wellbeing and reduced fatigue have been reported in trials with progestational agents. Sometimes early satiety will respond at least temporarily to the use of prokinetic agents (such as metoclopramide).

The metabolic management of patients should focus on down regulating the systemic inflammatory response to malignancy. Non-steroidal anti-inflammatory agents (such as ibuprofen 400 mg a day) along with peptic ulcer prophylaxis (such as omeprazole) can be used as long term treatment and have been combined successfully with progestational agents (as combination therapy to address reduced food intake). Eicosapentaenoic acid (EPA) is a natural component of fish oil and is known to down regulate proinflammatory cytokines and block the effects of tumour specific cachectic factors (for example, PIF). EPA (2 g a day) can be provided either as fish oil capsules or as a combination therapy by being incorporated in a high protein, high calorie oral sip feed (such as ProSure two cartons a day). This combination has been shown not only to arrest nutritional decline but also to improve patients' physical activity level.

Drugs with a direct anabolic effect have been suggested for the treatment of cachexia, and anabolic steroids have been shown to improve patients' weight without any apparent adverse effect. Tumours are well known to express growth factor receptors, and anabolic agents such as growth hormone are not used clinically because of anxieties about stimulating tumour growth.

Management of cachexia as outlined above may improve fatigue. If fatigue proves problematic or arises as a symptom in association with anaemia, recombinant erythropoietin may be of benefit. Recent evidence, however, has raised the issue of stimulation of tumour growth with erythropoietin in patients with head and neck cancer and this requires further evaluation. Fatigue may also be improved by anti-inflammatory strategies such as steroids or non-steroidal drugs. Finally, it is important to recognise that although some patients with cachexia can be

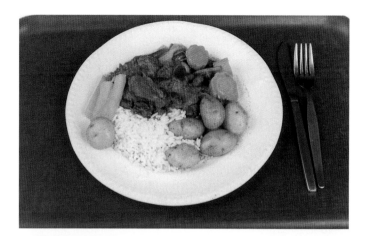

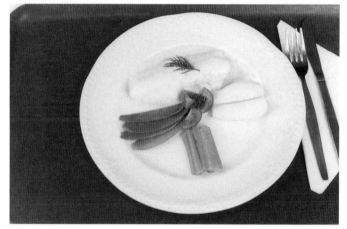

The size and appearance of meals may be as important as their nutritional value. Standard hospital meals (top) are generally unsuitable and should be replaced by smaller, more attractive helpings (bottom)

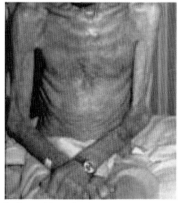

Patient with cachexia

improved, often the goals of intervention are to stabilise the situation or attenuate decline. Patients with limited energy reserves and capacity for physical activity, however, should be counselled to make most efficient use of the energy they have (with a focus on meal times and social interaction). Advice from occupational therapists and the provision of physical aids in the home may greatly enhance quality of life.

Patients should be encouraged to keep active to prevent secondary muscle wasting as a result of immobilisation

What can be expected from treatment of cachexia?

Cachexia is a multifactorial syndrome, the precise aetiology of which can vary from patient to patient. Thus it would be unreasonable to expect any single therapy to be effective in all patients. Improved nutritional status might increase physical function and thus quality of life and perhaps survival. Some patients might respond to combination therapy with weight stabilisation and resulting stable or improved physical function or quality of life.

The future

Combination therapy within the context of integrated care pathways promises better management of cachexia. At present, clinical trials are hampered by heterogeneity of patients, difficulty with defining end points, mild to moderate activity of combination regimens, loss of patients, and cost. Greater understanding of the complex pathophysiology of both cachexia and anorexia will hopefully provide new targets for drugs, which, in combination with better trial design, should lead to future progress.

Further reading

- Barber MD. The pathophysiology and treatment of cancer cachexia. *Nutr Clin Pract* 2002;17:203–9.
- Gordon JN, Green SR, Goggin PM. Cancer cachexia. *Q J Med* 2005;98:779–88.
- MacDonald N, Easson AM, Mazurak VC, Dunn GP, Baracos VE. Understanding and managing cancer cachexia. *J Am Coll Surg* 2003;197:143–61.
- Muscaritoli M, Bossola M, Aversa Z, Bellantone R, Rossi Fanelli F. Prevention and treatment of cancer cachexia: new insights into an old problem. *Eur J Cancer* 2006;42:31–41.
- Tisdale MJ. Molecular pathways leading to cancer cachexia. *Physiology* 2005;20:340–8.

7   Nausea and vomiting

Kathryn Mannix

Nausea and vomiting are related but separate symptoms; nausea is a sensation of the desire to vomit, which causes misery and withdrawal; vomiting is the action of expelling gastrointestinal contents via the mouth and is usually an involuntary reflex. Retching is a rhythmic contraction of the diaphragm, abdominal wall, and intercostal muscles, which propels vomit towards the mouth.

These are common symptoms in patients in palliative care, affecting up to 70% of people with advanced cancer and causing distress to considerable numbers of people with AIDS, heart failure, renal failure, and other life limiting conditions.

The symptom complex of nausea and vomiting is part of a brain stem reflex that has evolved to protect us from ingested poisons. Various triggers can stimulate nausea, and relief of nausea therefore requires identification of the trigger and treatment to remove the cause or to block central stimulation of receptors in the brain stem.

Managing nausea and vomiting

Adequate relief of these symptoms requires systematic assessment of the patient to diagnose the most likely cause(s). If the cause can be reversed—for example, with surgery to reverse gastrointestinal obstruction or measures to correct hypercalcaemia—then an antiemetic may be required only temporarily. In palliative care, however, the cause is often irreversible and a long term antiemetic strategy is required.

Prescribing antiemetic drugs is only part of such a strategy. Attention to the patient's understanding of the meaning of the symptoms, dealing with anxiety (which can cause or exacerbate nausea), and helping the patient to have realistic expectations about symptom management are important components of the strategy. Complementary therapies may have a role—for instance, there is good evidence for the efficacy of acupuncture in the management of nausea.

Antiemetics and other useful drugs

Pharmacological management of nausea and vomiting includes the use of drugs to block the emetogenic reflex in the brain stem (antiemetics), drugs to promote peristalsis in the upper gastrointestinal tract (prokinetic agents), drugs to reduce the volume of gastrointestinal secretions (antisecretory agents), and adjuvant drugs—for example, corticosteroids.

Choosing an antiemetic

Antiemetic drugs work by binding to specific receptor sites in the chemoreceptor trigger zone (CTZ) or vomiting centre (VC) in the brain stem. At each site there are several receptors; the more strongly the drug binds to its receptor, the more potent its antiemetic activity.

The most potent antiemetic at the CTZ is the dopamine antagonist haloperidol. At the VC, the non-sedating antihistamine cyclizine and the antimuscarinic hyoscine hydrobromide have similar efficacy, but the side effects of centrally acting antimuscarinics reduce their usefulness and makes cyclizine the drug of choice.

Levomepromazine is a phenothiazine with affinity for receptors at both the CTZ and the VC. Although its binding affinity is lower than cyclizine or haloperidol for the same receptors, it may be a useful broad spectrum antiemetic. It must

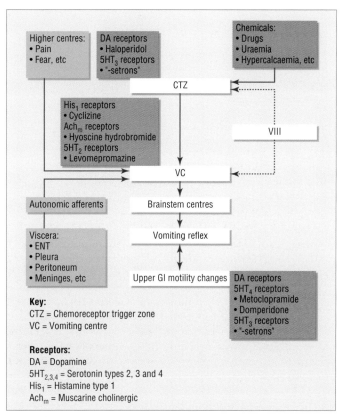

Triggers to nausea and vomiting: pathways, receptors, and recommended antiemetics

---

Drugs of use in the palliation of nausea and vomiting

Antiemetics
- Acting at CTZ: haloperidol, metoclopramide, levomepromazine
- Acting at vomiting centre: cyclizine, hyoscine hydrobromide, levomepromazine
- Acting on $5HT_3$ receptors (for nausea and vomiting induced only by chemotherapy, radiotherapy, or surgery): ondansetron, granisetron, tropisetron

Antisecretory agents
- Hyoscine hydrobromide
- Hyoscine butylbromide
- Octreotide

Prokinetic agents
- Metoclopramide
- Domperidone
- Cisapride*

Vestibular sedatives
- Cinnarizine
- Dimenhydrinate

Adjuvant drugs
- H_2 antagonists—for example, ranitidine, cimetidine
- Proton pump inhibitors—for example, omeprazole, lansoprazole
- Prostaglandin analogues—for example, misoprostol
- Corticosteroids
- Cannabinoids: nabilone

*Cardiotoxic: cisapride must be ordered on a named patient basis in the UK

There is no antiemetic role for $5HT_3$ antagonists, apart from their use in emesis induced by chemotherapy and possibly emesis after surgery

be used in low doses to avoid sedation and hypotension.

Metoclopramide has a lower affinity for CTZ dopamine receptors than haloperidol and so is less effective as an antiemetic. It has prokinetic activity because of its action on receptors in the gastrointestinal tract, and this is its major use in palliative care.

Steps to good management of symptoms

- Thorough assessment: history, examination, biochemistry, imaging, microbiology, and other investigations may all be required to establish a probable cause for nausea and/or vomiting
- Having identified a probable cause, determine what neurotransmitter receptors are likely to be involved
- Choose an antiemetic that is a specific antagonist to that neuroreceptor
- Give this antiemetic by a route that will ensure it will reach its target: in practical terms, this means avoiding the oral route (even in the absence of vomiting) until nausea has been settled for at least 24 hours
- Reassess. If nausea persists, there may be an additional trigger that has not been identified. Continue the first antiemetic while reassessing and introducing a second antiemetic acting at a different site in the brain stem
- Decide whether any of the triggers can be reversed. This depends both on the trigger and the patient's performance status or preference about other treatment options—for example, surgery, radiotherapy, dialysis
- Once nausea is controlled, plan how control will be maintained—for example, oral antiemetics, syringe driver, acupuncture, etc.

Non-drug approaches to palliation

Psychological techniques—Studies in people undergoing chemotherapy have shown that patients can learn progressive muscle relaxation and use mental imagery to increase their relaxation and reduce their nausea. Cognitive therapy has also been used to help to reduce the emotional distress arising from physical symptoms in advanced cancer. Hypnotherapy can help to reduce the sensation of nausea and the perceived duration of nausea.

Acupuncture and acupressure have both been shown to augment the effects of antiemetic drugs during chemotherapy and to reduce postoperative nausea and vomiting. Transcutaneous electrical nerve stimulation (TENS) can be used as an alternative to traditional acupuncture needles at the P6 acupuncture point, and this is more practical for patients to use themselves.

Management of specific nausea and vomiting syndromes

Gastric stasis

Reduction in gastric emptying may be caused by opioids, mucosal inflammation (NSAIDs, stress, tumour), anticholinergic drugs (including side effects of tricyclic antidepressants and antipsychotics), raised intra-abdominal pressure (ascites, hepatomegaly), or occasionally by encroachment of tumour on the gastric outlet (such as gastroduodenal tumours, mass in head of pancreas).

Autonomic failure may be a feature of end stage cancer, Parkinson's disease, diabetes, and AIDS and can allow pooling of gastric secretions in a patulous stomach, with regurgitation and posseting.

> **Gastric emptying is reduced in the presence of nausea. Don't assume that oral drugs will work, even if there is no vomiting**

Steps to good management
- Carry out a thorough assessment
- Determine which neurotransmitter receptors are involved
- Choose an antiemetic for the specific neuroreceptor
- Choose the relevant route of administration
- Reassess to identify any additional triggers
- Decide whether any of triggers can be reversed
- Plan how to maintain control

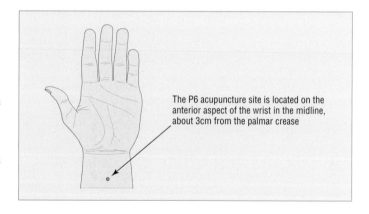

The P6 acupuncture site is located on the anterior aspect of the wrist in the midline, about 3cm from the palmar crease

---

Common chemical causes of nausea and vomiting
- Opioids (30% of patients at introduction of opioids)
- Hypercalcaemia
- Uraemia (urinary tract obstruction, renal failure, heart failure)
- Chemotherapy

Assessment

There is little nausea because the stomach is designed to stretch. Large volume vomits are characteristic; as the stomach distends the patient may experience acid reflux through the distended cardia, hiccups triggered by diaphragmatic irritation, a feeling of bloating, and early satiation after taking small amounts of food or drink. Vomiting usually relieves these symptoms, and the vomit may contain undigested food eaten many hours earlier.

Management

Anticholinergic drugs must be discontinued if at all possible. Prokinetic drugs may restore gastric emptying if the lumen is patent and the autonomic nerves are intact, but they may cause colic if there is an upper gastrointestinal obstruction. In normal circumstances, using a proton pump inhibitor or H_2 blocker can reduce the volume of gastric secretions, and parenteral administration can help some patients with obstruction. Ingested air can be de-foamed with dimethicone (tablets or compounded with an antacid).

Occasionally a tube may be necessary to decompress the stomach: a venting PEG (percutaneous endoscopic gastrostomy) tube may be more acceptable than a nasogastric tube. A dual lumen PEG, with a jejunal extension, may be used to aspirate from the stomach and to deliver enteral fluids to the jejunum, preventing dehydration.

Gastrointestinal obstruction

Malignant obstruction of the gastrointestinal tract may be due to occlusion of the lumen by tumour or distortion of gut and mesentery by tumour, or may be functional due to a failure of normal peristalsis. Obstruction may be partial or complete and may develop gradually with self resolving episodes of partial obstruction preceding a complete obstruction. The treatment of choice for a single level of occlusion is surgery, but when the patient is unfit for surgery, or when there are multiple levels of obstruction, an alternative treatment regimen is necessary to palliate symptoms of nausea, vomiting, colic, abdominal distension, and peritoneal pain.

The amount of vomiting depends on the level of obstruction, with more proximal upper gastrointestinal obstruction causing larger volume vomiting. If the level of obstruction is beyond the mid-jejunum, the mucosa of the upper gastrointestinal tract can continue to absorb fluids from the lumen. This reduces the volume of intestinal contents and, in turn, reduces the gut distension that triggers nausea and colic. Thus, vomiting is less frequent and of smaller volumes with more distal obstruction.

Nausea is triggered by distension of the bowel lumen, stimulating the vomiting centre via autonomic afferents. The antiemetics of choice are cyclizine or levomepromazine, and a non-oral route is required to ensure its activity. Absorption of bacterial toxins from a stagnant or ischaemic area of obstructed bowel can also trigger nausea via the chemoreceptor trigger zone: this situation would require the use of a CTZ antiemetic in addition to cyclizine, and haloperidol is the drug of choice, again by a non-oral route.

Dehydration can complicate proximal obstruction, as intestinal secretions are vomited along with any ingested fluids. The volume of intestinal secretion can be reduced by using antisecretory agents: hyoscine butylbromide and octreotide have both been used successfully to reduce pancreatic and upper gastrointestinal secretions. Hyoscine butylbromide also reduces colic. The inhibition of gastric secretions is described above. Dehydration can cause neuromuscular irritability and thirst: good mouth care is essential. If parenteral fluids are required, subcutaneous fluids are well tolerated and can be administered

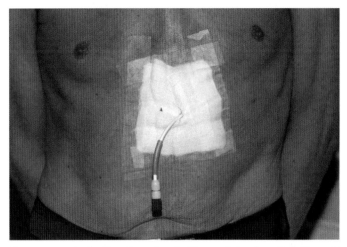

Gastrostomy tube feeding. Reproduced with permission from Dr P Marazzi/ Science Photy Library

Palliation of symptoms of intestinal obstruction

Drug/dose	Actions	Comments
Cyclizine 150 mg/24 hours sc infusion may require addition of haloperidol 1.5–3 mg sc once a day	Acts on vomiting centre	Nausea is controllable but vomiting will persist in total obstruction
Haloperidol 1.5–3 mg sc once a day	Acts on CTZ	
Hyoscine butylbromide 60–200 mg/24 hours	Reduces motility and secretions	Both drugs reduce distension reducing nausea and colic
Octreotide 300–1200 µg/24 hours	Reduces secretions	
Levomepromazine 6.25–25 mg/24 hours	Acts on VC and CTZ, useful second line antiemetic	Sedating at higher doses

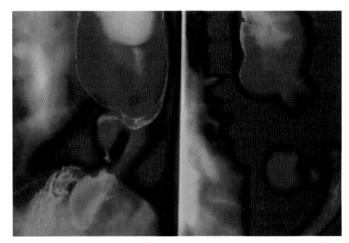

Coloured x-rays showing a healthy human intestine, and the same intestine which has become obstructed. Reproduced with permission from Bsip Vem/Science Photo Library

at home if necessary.

Nasogastric intubation does not relieve nausea and may exacerbate nausea by irritating the pharynx. Use of a nasogastric tube to empty the stomach before surgery is entirely appropriate, however, and occasionally it may be appropriate to use intermittently. This depends entirely on the individual patient. In patients with high obstruction, a venting PEG may palliate frequent vomiting.

It is important that patients and families understand that intermittent vomiting is likely to continue despite the control of nausea and colic. Patients with intestinal obstruction, however, may still enjoy the pleasure of eating and drinking; those with low obstruction will be able to absorb some nutrition in this way. Eating and drinking as desired should be encouraged.

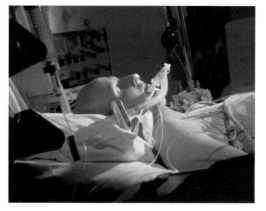

Man in cardiac intensive care on a respirator and linked to a nasogastric tube. Reproduced with permission from Deep Light Productions/Science Photo Library

Drug induced nausea and vomiting

Many drugs can cause nausea and vomiting. If the offending drug cannot be withdrawn, then identification of the way in which nausea is triggered should be part of symptom management—for example, gastroprotectant treatment for drug induced gastritis, or an antiemetic acting at the CTZ for chemically induced nausea.

Emesis induced by chemotherapy is a particular challenge. Early nausea is mediated by $5HT_3$ receptors in the gastrointestinal tract, and possibly in the CTZ, and is best palliated by using antiemetic protocols recommended by the oncology team. This will include the use of specific $5HT_3$ antagonists for the more emetogenic drugs, such as platinum and ipfosfamide. Regimens may also include corticosteroids and sedative drugs. Delayed nausea after chemotherapy continues to be a problem, and investigation of novel antiemetic agents is awaited.

Other considerations

Once nausea is present, gastric emptying will be slow and oral drugs may be unreliably absorbed from the gastrointestinal tract. In patients with nausea or vomiting, or both, it is therefore important to consider the best way in which to continue any necessary medications.

Opioid analgesics can be given by injection (a continuous, subcutaneous infusion is usually more comfortable and convenient than regular intermittent injections), suppository, transdermal patch, and transmucosal lozenge, according to the drug and dose required. It is important to ensure that the dose is modified appropriately in conversion from the oral to an alternative route (see chapter 2).

Vomiting is tiring, and patients may need to be encouraged to rest. Practical considerations include providing suitably large vomit bowls, particularly in gastric stasis or high obstruction, when volumes of vomit can be big. Mouth care is an important component of ensuring comfort for people who are vomiting or who are dehydrated.

Causes of nausea and vomiting induced by drugs

Mechanism	Drugs
Chemical trigger at CTZ in brainstem	Opioids, cytotoxics, digoxin, imidazoles, anticoagulants, antibiotics
Gastrointestinal irritation	Non-steroidal anti-inflammatory drugs, iron supplements, antibiotics, cytotoxics
Gastric stasis	Tricyclics, opioids, phenothiazines, antimuscarinics

Mouth care is a vital part of comfort management for people who are dehydrated or vomiting

Further reading
- Doyle D, Hanks GW, Cherny N, Calman K, eds. *The Oxford textbook of palliative medicine*. 3rd ed. Oxford: Oxford University Press, 2004.

8   Constipation, diarrhoea, and intestinal obstruction

Nigel Sykes, Carla Ripamonti, Eduardo Bruera, Debra Gordon

Constipation

Prevalence
Constipation is the infrequent and difficult passage of small hard faeces. About 80% of patients in palliative care will require laxatives.

Constipation

Definition
- Infrequent hard stools

Associated symptoms	**Symptoms of complications**
- Flatulence	- Anorexia
- Bloating	- Overflow diarrhoea
- Abdominal pain	- Confusion
- Feeling of incomplete evacuation	- Nausea and vomiting
	- Urinary dysfunction

Assessment

History

The frequency and consistency of stools, nausea, vomiting, abdominal pain, distension and discomfort, mobility, diet, and previous bowel habit should be determined. In patients with a history of diarrhoea, true diarrhoea should be distinguished from overflow due to faecal impaction.

Examination

Constipation must be distinguished from obstruction due to tumour. Faecal masses are indentable, mobile, and rarely tender and may be palpable in the colon. In contrast, tumour masses are usually hard, fixed, and often tender. In obstruction, auscultation of the abdomen may reveal high pitched tinkling bowel sounds.

Digital examination may show an empty rectum or stoma in constipation—hard stools can lie higher in the bowel. However, 90% of impactions occur in the rectum, so examination can distinguish overflow from true diarrhoea.

Investigation with radiography

If the diagnosis of constipation is still unclear, despite an accurate history and examination, supine and erect abdominal radiography will show the characteristic meniscal appearance of gas and fluid filled bowel.

> Assessment of constipation must include establishing in what way the present pattern of bowel movements is different from the normal pattern and a physical examination, including general observation, abdominal palpation, and rectal or stomal examination

Management of constipation

The most important causes of constipation are immobility, poor fluid and dietary intake, and drugs, particularly opioids. Good general symptom control will minimise the first three of these, but most patients will require laxatives. The aim of laxative therapy is to achieve comfortable defecation, rather than any particular frequency of bowel movement. The choice of laxative depends on the nature of the stools, acceptability to the patient, and cost. Dose should be titrated against individual response. Clinically it is useful to divide laxatives into two groups:
- Predominantly softening
- Predominantly stimulating peristalsis

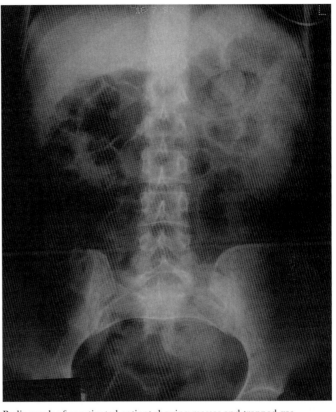

Radiograph of constipated patient showing masses and trapped gas

---

Causes of constipation

Caused by cancer
- Hypercalcaemia
- Intra-abdominal or pelvic disease
- Compression of spinal cord
- Cauda equina syndrome
- Depression

Caused by treatment
- Opioids
- Antiemetics—cyclizine, ondansetron
- Anticholinergics—antispasmodics, antidepressants, neuroleptics
- Aluminium salts
- Non-steroidal anti-inflammatory drugs

Associated with debility
- Weakness
- Inactivity or bed rest
- Poor nutrition
- Poor fluid intake
- Confusion
- Inability to reach the toilet

Concurrent disorders
- Haemorrhoids
- Anal fissure
- Endocrine dysfunction

Vicious cycle of constipation associated with opioid analgesics

Systematic reviews suggest most laxatives have similar effectiveness, but in constipation related to opioid use, doses and adverse effects can both be minimised by the use of a combination of softening and stimulant laxatives.

Predominantly softening laxatives
Surfactant laxatives, such as poloxamer and docusate, act as detergents, increasing water penetration and hence softening the stools. They are available in combination with the peristalsis stimulator dantron.

Osmotic laxatives—Lactulose is popular but can cause bloating and flatulence and is too sweet for some patients. Saline laxatives, such as magnesium sulphate or hydroxide, have a mixed osmotic and stimulant mode of action and at higher doses can be strongly purgative. Magnesium hydroxide in combination with the lubricant softener liquid paraffin (now rarely used on its own) is a cheaper alternative to lactulose. Macrogols (polyethylene glycols) are administered with fluid, and they do not therefore draw further fluid from the body into the bowel. These drugs are now commonly used.

Non-absorbable fluid is provided by polyethylene glycol. The volume required can be difficult for ill patients.

Bulk forming agents are stool normalisers rather than true laxatives. They are less helpful in patients with cancer because of the volume of water required, their unproved efficacy in severe constipation, and the possibility of worsening an incipient obstruction.

Stimulant laxatives
These drugs stimulate the myenteric plexus to induce peristalsis and reduce net absorption of water and electrolytes in the colon. The latency of action is 6–12 hours. They can cause abdominal colic and severe purgation. Giving a stimulant in combination with a softening laxative may reduce colic. The most popular stimulants are senna and dantron. Patients given dantron may experience reddish discoloration of the urine and perianal rash, particularly in incontinent patients. (Dantron preparations are reserved for patients who have advanced cancer.)

Rectal laxatives
Suppositories or enemas are sometimes necessary but should never accompany an inadequate prescription of an oral laxative. They are appropriate for treating faecal impaction and for conditions such as spinal cord compression, when long term use may be necessary.

Diarrhoea

Diarrhoea is much less common than constipation in patients with advanced disease, affecting less than 10% of patients with cancer admitted to hospital or palliative care units.

Causes
The most common cause of diarrhoea in patients with advanced disease is use of laxatives. Patients may use laxatives erratically; some wait until they become constipated and then use high doses of laxatives, with resultant rebound diarrhoea. Among elderly patients admitted to hospital with non-malignant disease, constipation with faecal impaction and overflow accounts for over half the cases of diarrhoea.

Management
The underlying cause should be investigated, but relief is generally achieved with non-specific antidiarrhoeal agents—loperamide (up to 16 mg daily) or codeine (10–60 mg every four hours). Codeine may cause central effects, but these are rare

> A distended rectum or colon can be a major cause of agitation and pain in a dying patient. Evacuation of the rectum or colon with suppositories alone or with an enema can give complete relief. The use of opioids to treat the pain of constipation only makes the constipation, and ultimately the pain, worse and a vicious cycle ensues

Questions to guide choice of rectal laxative
- Is the rectum or stoma full?
- Is the stool hard or soft?
- Is the rectum or stoma empty but the colon full?
- Are the rectum and colon both full?
- Does the patient have rectal sensation?
- Does the patient have normal anal tone?
- If a cord lesion is present what is the level?

Choices of rectal laxative
- Bisacodyl suppository—Evacuates stools from rectum or stoma; for colonic inertia
- Glycerine suppository—Softens stools in rectum or stoma
- Phosphate enema—Evacuates stools from lower bowel
- Arachis oil enema—Softens hard impacted stools

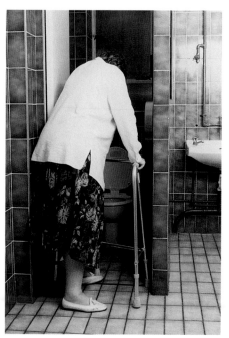

Access and ability to get to a toilet may be more important in patients with constipation than supply of laxatives

Causes of diarrhoea in patients with advanced disease
- Drugs
  Laxatives
  Antibiotics
  Antacids
  Chemotherapy
  (5-fluorouracil)
- Diet
- Tumour
  Colon or rectum
  Pelvic
  Pancreatic (islet cell)
  Carcinoid
  Fistula
- Radiotherapy
- Intestinal obstruction (including faecal impaction)
- Concurrent disease, such as inflammatory bowel disease
- Malabsorption
  Pancreatic carcinoma
  Gastrectomy
  Ileal resection
  Colectony
- Infection

with loperamide.

Rarely, patients with intractable diarrhoea may require a subcutaneous infusion of octreotide; the usual indication is a high effluent volume from a stoma. Diarrhoea due to malabsorption, often associated with pancreatic cancer, responds to pancreatic enzyme supplementation.

Intestinal obstruction

Epidemiology and pathophysiology
Intestinal obstruction is any process preventing the movement of bowel contents, thus leading to the partial or complete blocking of faeces and gas through the intestinal passage. Malignant intestinal obstruction (MIO) is common in patients with abdominal or pelvic cancers, with the highest incidence ranging from 5.5% to 51% in women with ovarian carcinoma, in whom it is a major cause of mortality. MIO occurs in 4.4% to 28.4% in patients with colorectal cancer and has been reported in patients with other advanced cancers, ranging from 3% to 15% of cases. Intestinal obstruction can be partial or complete, single or multiple, and due to benign causes (ranging from 6.1% in ovarian and other gynaecological cancers to 48% in colorectal cancer) or malignant causes. The small bowel is more commonly affected than the large bowel (61% *v* 33%) and both are affected in over a fifth of patients.

Several mechanisms may be involved in the onset of MIO, and there is variability in both presentation and aetiology. At least three factors occur in bowel obstruction:

- Accumulation of gastric, pancreatic, and biliary secretions that are a potent stimulus for further intestinal secretions
- Decreased absorption of water and sodium from the intestinal lumen
- Increased secretion of water and sodium into the lumen as distension increases.

Loss of fluids and electrolytes results in breakdown of the sequence of secretion and reabsorption in the gastrointestinal tract. Secretions accumulate in the bowel above the obstruction. The volume of secretions tends to increase after intestinal distension and the consequent increase in the surface area, thus producing a vicious circle of secretion-distension-secretion.

The vicious circle represented by distension-secretion-motor hyperactivity exacerbates the clinical picture, producing intraluminal hypertension and epithelial damage. Epithelial damage generates an inflammatory response and the release of prostaglandins, potent secretagogues, either by a direct effect on enterocytes or enteric nervous reflex. Furthermore, vasoactive intestinal polypeptide (VIP) might be released into the portal and peripheral circulation. This mediates local intestinal and systemic pathophysiological changes accompanying small intestinal obstruction, such as hyperaemia and oedema of the intestinal wall and accumulation of fluid in the lumen due to its stimulating effects.

Signs, symptoms, diagnosis, and investigations
In patients with cancer, compression of the bowel lumen develops slowly and often remains partial. As a consequence of the partial or complete occlusion to the lumen and/or dysmotility, the accumulation of the unabsorbed secretions produces nausea, vomiting, intermittent or complete constipation, pain, and colicky activity to surmount the obstacle that causes colicky pain. Abdominal distension may be absent in high obstruction—that is, of the duodenum or proximal jejunum—and when the bowel is "plastered" down by extensive mesenteric spread.

Pathophysiological mechanisms of malignant intestinal obstruction (MIO)

Mechanical obstruction is caused by:
- Extrinsic occlusion of the lumen due to an enlargement of the primary tumour or recurrence, mesenteric and omental masses, abdominal or pelvic adhesions (benign or malignant), postirradiation fibrosis; postirradiation intestinal damage
- Intraluminal occlusion of the lumen due to neoplastic mass, polypoidal lesions, or annular tumoral dissemination
- Intramural occlusion of the lumen due to intestinal linitis plastica

Functional obstruction (or adynamic ileus) is caused by intestinal motility disorders as a result of:
- Tumour infiltration of the mesentery or bowel muscle and nerves (carcinomatosis), malignant involvement of the coeliac plexus
- Paraneoplastic neuropathy in patients with lung cancer
- Chronic intestinal pseudo-obstruction (CIP) mainly due to diabetes mellitus, previous gastric surgery, neurological disorders, or drugs such as opioids
- Paraneoplastic pseudo-obstruction

Other causes such as inflammatory oedema, faecal impaction, constipating drugs such as opioids, anticholinergics, belladonna alkaloids, antidepressants, vinca alkaloids, etc), and dehydration can contribute to the development of intestinal obstruction or worsen the clinical picture

---

Depletion of water and salt in the lumen is the most important "toxic factor" in bowel obstruction

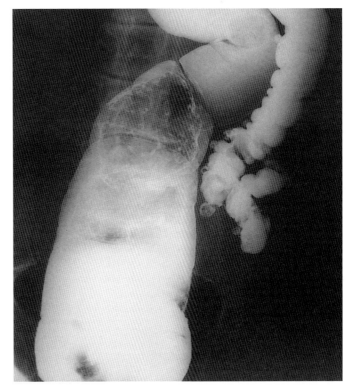

Radiograph showing megacolon secondary to rectal carcinoma

Common symptoms in cancer patients with MIO

Vomiting	Intermittent or continuous	Develops early and in large amounts in gastric, duodenal, and small bowel obstruction and develops later in large bowel obstruction	Biliary vomiting is almost odourless and indicates an obstruction in the upper part of the abdomen. The presence of bad smelling and faeculent vomiting can be the first sign of an ileal or colonic obstruction
Nausea	Intermittent or continuous		
Colicky pain	Variable intensity and localization due to distension proximal to the obstruction secondary to gas and fluid accumulation most of which is produced by the gut; present in 75% of patients	If it is intense, periumbilical, and occurring at brief intervals, it may be an indication of an obstruction at the jejunum-ileal level. In large bowel obstruction the pain is less intense, deeper, and occurs at longer intervals	Overall acute pain that begins intensely and becomes stronger, or pain that is specifically localised, may be a symptom of a perforation or an ileal or colonic strangulation. Pain that increases with palpation may be due to peritoneal irritation
Continuous pain	Variable intensity and localisation; present in 90% of patients	Due to abdominal distension, tumour mass, and/or hepatomegaly	
Dry mouth		Due to severe dehydration and metabolic alterations but mostly due to the use of drugs with anticholinergic properties and poor mouth care	
Constipation	Intermittent or complete	In case of complete obstruction there is no evacuation of faeces and no flatus	In case of partial obstruction the symptom is intermittent
Overflow diarrhoea		Result of bacterial liquefaction of faecal material	

Gastrointestinal symptoms caused by the sequence of distension-secretion-motor activity of the obstructed bowel occur in different combinations and intensity depending on the site of obstruction. The symptoms referred to by the patient should be monitored daily. Vomiting can be evaluated in terms of quantity, quality, and number of daily episodes. Numerical or verbal scales can be used to assess other symptoms, such as nausea, pain, dry mouth, drowsiness, dyspnoea, hunger, thirst, etc.

When a patient with cancer presents with suspected bowel obstruction, a full assessment should be performed. Various radiological investigations can be performed in patients with signs and symptoms of MIO. There is no point in proceeding with any of these, however, if the patient is too ill or has declined surgery.

Management of intestinal obstruction

In patients with advanced cancer MIO is rarely an emergency event and intestinal strangulation is uncommon, thus there is time to evaluate the most suitable therapeutic intervention for each patient. In the face of a clearly incurable situation, decision making has to be a careful, balanced process with the individual patient at the centre.

Curative or palliative surgery

Surgical intervention should be considered in all patients with MIO, though it should not routinely be undertaken in patients with advanced and end stage cancer who do not have a benign cause of occlusion. Generally surgery will be appropriate only in selected patients such as those with mechanical obstruction and/or limited tumour bulk, single site of obstruction, and no or minimal ascites, and those with a reasonable chance of further response to anticancer therapy.

If surgery is being considered, you should assess whether:

- Palliative surgery is technically feasible?
- The patient is likely to benefit from surgery not only in terms of survival but above all in terms of quality of life?

Published data show that in patients with advanced cancer, the operative mortality is 9–40% and complication rates vary from 9–90%. The type of obstruction (partial v complete) and the method of surgical treatment (bypass v resection and reanastomosis) have no measurable effect on the outcome. As

Assessment in patients with suspected MIO

- Other causes of nausea, vomiting, and constipation
- Metabolic abnormalities
- Type and doses of drugs
- Nutritional and hydration status
- Abdominal masses
- Ascites
- Faecal impaction, examine rectum or stoma

Radiological investigations

Plain radiography
To document the dilated loops of bowel, air-fluid interfaces, or both

Contrast radiography
Investigations help to evaluate dysmotility and partial obstruction and to define the site and extent of obstruction. Erect abdomen gastrografin (diatrizoate meglumine) is useful in such cases; moreover, it often provides excellent visualisation of proximal obstructions and can reduce luminal oedema and help to resolve partial obstructions. Contrast studies of the stomach, gastric outlet, and small bowel can help to distinguish obstructions from metastases, radiation injury, or adhesions. The diagnosis of a motility disorder is revealed by the slow passage of contrast through undilated bowel with no demonstrable point of obstruction Retrograde, transrectal contrast studies (barium or water soluble medium enema) can rule out and diagnose isolated or concomitant obstruction of the large bowel
Often the most efficient and practical assessment is computed tomography of abdomen and pelvis with appropriate oral and/or rectal gastrografin

Computed tomography
Abdominal CT with contrast is useful to evaluate the global extent of disease, to perform staging, and to assist in the choice of surgical, endoscopic, or simple pharmacological palliative intervention for the management of the obstruction

Endoscopy
Once a site of obstruction is identified in either the gastric outlet or colon, endoscopic studies may be helpful to evaluate the exact cause of the obstruction. This is particularly important when endoscopic treatment approaches, such as stent placement, are considered

recently published results are no better than those published in the past, improvements in surgical techniques and perioperative care seem not to influence the outcome. Results may reflect the poor clinical condition of patients at the time of surgery. Although the surgical literature reports the survival of the obstructed patients operated on, most publications do not describe the outcome assessment of quality of life, postoperative complications, length of admission, control of symptoms, and patient's comfort.

Prognostic criteria are needed to help doctors to select patients who are likely to benefit from surgical intervention. Based on retrospective data, several authors have derived clinical parameters that indicate low likelihood of clinical benefit from surgical management of intestinal obstruction. Patients with two or more poor prognostic factors can have an operative mortality of 44% compared with 13% among those with one or no risk factors.

Surgical palliation in patients with advanced cancer is a complex issue, and the decision to proceed with surgery must be carefully evaluated for each individual.

Self expanding metallic stents
Stents are an option in patients with malignant obstruction of the gastric outlet, proximal small bowel, and colon. The stents may be useful in the management of patients who are at surgical risk or in those presenting with large bowel obstruction in which decompression by a stent allows treatment of coexisting medical complications to enable surgery to be carried out at a later date, after staging of the disease and an optimal colonic preparation. However, their usefulness in patients with end stage cancer has to be evaluated.

Venting procedures
In inoperable patients, the usual treatment consists of drainage with a nasogastric tube associated with parenteral hydration. A nasogastric tube can cause great discomfort to the patient and several complications (for instance, erosion of the nasal cartilage, otitis media, aspiration pneumonia, oesophagitis and bleeding). Therefore, it should be considered a temporary measure to reduce the gastric distension when drugs are ineffective for symptom control or when gastrostomy cannot be carried out. If continued drainage is required, operative or percutaneous endoscopic gastrostomy are much better for decompression of the GI tract.

Pharmacological palliative treatment
The pharmacological management of intestinal obstruction due to advanced cancer focuses on the treatment of nausea, vomiting, pain, and other symptoms without the use of venting procedures. Dose and choice of drug should be tailored to the individual patient. Most MIO patients cannot use the oral route, and alternative routes should be considered. Continuous subcutaneous infusion of drugs with a portable syringe driver allows the parenteral administration of different drug combinations, produces minimal discomfort for the patient, and is easy to use at home. If a central venous catheter has previously been inserted, this can be used to administer drugs for symptom control. Rectal and sublingual administration can occasionally be used. Finally, some drugs, such as fentanyl, buprenorphine, and scopolamine, may be also administered transdermally.

Pain
Various opioids, administered via different routes according to the WHO guidelines, are the most effective drugs for the

Contraindications to surgery
Obstruction secondary to cancer

Absolute contraindication
- Intestinal motility problems due to diffuse intraperitoneal carcinomatosis
- Ascites requiring frequent paracentesis
- Diffuse palpable intra-abdominal masses
- Multiple partial bowel obstruction with prolonged passage time on radiograph examination
- Recent laparotomy that showed that further corrective surgery was not possible
- Previous abdominal surgery that showed diffuse metastatic cancer

Relative contraindication
- Widespread tumour
- Patients aged >65 with cachexia
- Low serum albumin concentration
- Previous radiotherapy of the abdomen or pelvis
- Poor nutritional status
- Liver metastases, distant metastases, pleural effusion, or pulmonary metastases producing symptoms
- Raised blood urea and creatinine concentrations, raised alkaline phosphatase activity, advanced tumour stage, short diagnosis to obstruction interval
- Poor performance status
- Extra-abdominal metastases producing symptoms difficult to control (for example, dyspnoea)

> **Consent to palliative surgery should include discussion of the surgical risks, complications, and alternatives such as pharmacological management for symptom control and stenting and venting procedures**

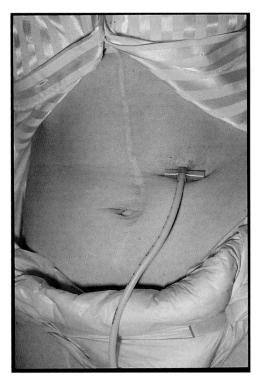

Percutaneous endoscopic gastrostomy

Drugs used for treatment of nausea, vomiting and pain
- Opioid analgesics
- Antiemetics
- Antisecretory drugs to decrease the GI secretions

ABC of palliative care

management of abdominal continuous and colicky pain associated with bowel obstruction. Anticholinergic drugs such as hyoscine butylbromide, hyoscine hydrobromide, or glycopyrolate, can be added to opioids in the presence of colicky pain if the opioids alone are not effective.

Nausea and vomiting

The box shows various drugs and doses used to control nausea and vomiting in patients with bowel obstruction according to first principles and available data. Vomiting can be managed with two different pharmacological approaches:

- Drugs such as anticholinergics and/or octreotide, which reduce gastrointestinal secretions
- Antiemetics acting on the central nervous system, alone or in association with drugs to reduce gastrointestinal secretions.

Hyoscine butylbromide is often used for both vomiting and colicky pain by some palliative care centres. Dry mouth is reported to be the most severe side effect. Sucking ice cubes and drinking small sips of water along with regular mouth care can help. Octreotide, a synthetic analogue of somatostatin that has a more potent biological activity and a longer half life, has also been used to manage the symptoms of bowel obstruction. Somatostatin and its analogues have been shown to inhibit the release and activity of gastrointestinal hormones, modulate gastrointestinal function by reducing gastric acid secretion, slow intestinal motility, decrease bile flow, increase mucous production, and reduce splanchnic blood flow. It reduces gastrointestinal contents and increases absorption of water and electrolytes at intracellular level, via cAMP and calcium regulation. The inhibitory effect of octreotide on both peristalsis and secretions reduces bowel distension and the secretion of water and sodium by the intestinal epithelium, thereby reducing vomiting and pain. The drug may therefore break the vicious circle represented by secretion, distension, and contractile hyperactivity.

Octreotide is considerably more effective and faster than hyoscine butylbromide in reducing the amount of gastrointestinal secretions in patients with a nasogastric tube and in reducing the intensity of nausea and the number of vomiting episodes in patients without a nasogastric tube. Moreover octreotide may prevent the development of irreversible bowel obstruction in patients with recurrent episodes of obstruction. Octreotide is an expensive drug and its cost to benefit ratio should be carefully considered, especially for prolonged treatment. The cost of the drug, however, should be interpreted in the widest possible sense—that is, if the use of a drug results in a more rapid improvement of gastrointestinal symptoms, which potentially limits the bed stay or the admission to an inpatient unit, in addition to a better quality of life for the patient.

Among the antiemetics haloperidol is the drug of choice by palliative care specialists. Haloperidol can be combined with hyoscine butylbromide and opioid analgesia in the same syringe. Metoclopramide is the drug of choice in functional intestinal obstruction; it is not recommended in patients with complete bowel obstruction because it may increase nausea, vomiting, and colicky pain. Other antiemetics are the butyrophenones, antihistaminic-antiemetics, and phenothiazines.

Parenteral corticosteroids are sometimes used for additional symptomatic relief of bowel obstruction. This is a difficult area to study and currently there is a lack of good evidence for the most appropriate role and dosing regimen.

Hydration and total parenteral nutrition (TPN)

In patients with inoperable intestinal obstruction the amount of

Palliation of symptoms of intestinal obstruction

Drug/dose	Actions	Comments
Cyclizine 150 mg/24 h subcutaneous infusion may require addition of haloperidol	Acts on vomiting centre	Nausea is controllable but vomiting will persist in total obstruction
Haloperidol 1.5-3 mg subcutaneous once daily	Acts on chemoreceptor trigger zone	
Hyoscine butylbromide 60-200 mg/24 h	Reduces motility and secretions	Both drugs reduce distension, reducing nausea, vomiting and colic
Octreotide 300-1200 µg/24 h	Reduces secretions	
Levomepromazine 6.25-25 mg/24 h	Acts on vomiting centre and chemoreceptor trigger zone; useful second line antiemetic	Sedating at higher doses

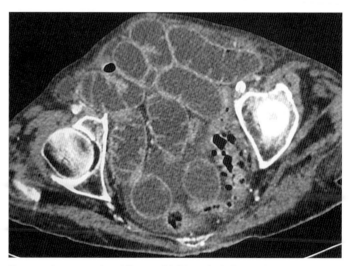

Computed tomography of "inoperable" intestinal obstruction

34

fluid administered should be assessed carefully. High levels of intravenous and subcutaneous fluids may result in more bowel secretions, thus it is necessary to keep a balance between the efficacy of the treatment and the side effects such as increased vomiting, abdominal distension, and pain. The intensity of dry mouth and thirst are independent of the quantity of parenteral and oral hydration. The intensity of nausea, however, is considerably lower in patients treated with more than 1 litre/day of parenteral fluids. Hydration can also improve fatigue and delirium in selected patients. Intravenous hydration can be difficult and uncomfortable for some patients with end stage cancer. Hypodermoclysis is a simple technique for rehydration that offers many advantages over the intravenous route, especially in patients at home. The role of TPN in the management of patients with inoperable bowel obstruction is controversial. No data are available on the survival rates or quality of life in patients with advanced cancer treated with this. TPN may be considered a futile treatment or an acceptable means of maintaining patient autonomy; hence, while it is not commonly indicated, it will remain a decision made on an individual basis.

Further reading

- Ripamonti C, Bruera E, eds. *Gastrointestinal symptoms in advanced cancer patients*. Oxford: Oxford University Press, 2002.

9 Depression, anxiety, and confusion

Mari Lloyd-Williams

Despite many advances in the palliation and management of the symptoms of advanced cancer, the assessment and management of psychological and psychiatric symptoms are still poor.

A common misapprehension is to assume that depression and anxiety represent understandable reactions to incurable illness. When cure is not possible, the analytical approach we adopt to physical and psychological signs and symptoms is often forgotten. This error of approach and the lack of diagnostic importance given to major and minor symptoms of depression result in underdiagnosis and undertreatment of psychiatric disorder.

Psychological adjustment reactions after diagnosis or relapse often include fear, sadness, perplexity, and anger. These usually resolve within a few weeks with the help of the patient's own personal resources, family support, and professional care. However, 10–20% of patients will develop formal psychiatric disorders that require specific evaluation and management in addition to general support.

Causes

Depression and anxiety are usually reactions to the losses and threats of the medical illness. Other risk factors often contribute.

Confusion usually reflects an organic mental disorder from one or more causes, often worsened by bewilderment and distress, discomfort or pain, and being in unfamiliar surroundings with unfamiliar carers. Elderly patients with impaired memory, hearing, or sight are especially at risk. Unfortunately, reversible causes of confusion are underdiagnosed, and this causes unnecessary distress in patients and families.

Clinical features

Depression and anxiety

These are broad terms that cover a continuum of emotional states. It is not always possible on the basis of a single interview to distinguish self limiting distress, which forms a natural part of the adjustment process, from the psychiatric syndromes of depressive illness and anxiety state, which need specific treatment. Borderline cases are common, and both the somatic and psychological symptoms of depression and anxiety can make diagnosis difficult.

Somatic symptoms—Depression may manifest itself as intractable pain, while anxiety can manifest itself as nausea or dyspnoea. Such symptoms may seem disproportionate to the medical pathology and respond poorly to medical treatments.

Psychological symptoms—Although these might seem understandable, they differ in severity, duration, and quality from "normal" distress. Depressed patients seem to loathe themselves, over and above loathing their disease. A useful analogy is that the patient who is sad blames the illness for how they feel, whereas a patient who is depressed blames themselves for their illness. This expresses itself through guilt about being ill and a burden to others, pervasive loss of interest and pleasure, and hopelessness about the future. Attempted suicide or requests for euthanasia, however rational they might seem, invariably indicate clinical depression. It is important that such thoughts are elicited—for example, by asking "have you ever felt so bad that you wanted to harm or kill yourself?"

Losses and threats of major illness

- Knowledge of a life threatening diagnosis, prognostic uncertainty, fears about dying and death
- Uncontrolled physical symptoms such as pain and nausea
- Unwanted effects of medical and surgical treatments
- Loss of functional capacity, loss of independence, enforced changes in role
- Spiritual questions, uncertainty and distress
- Practical issues such as finance, work, housing
- Changes in relationships, concern for dependants
- Changes in body image, sexual dysfunction, infertility

It is important to recognise psychiatric disorders because, if untreated, they add to the suffering of patients and their friends and relatives

---

Risk factors for anxiety and depression

- Organic mental disorders
- Poorly controlled physical symptoms
- Poor relationships and communication between staff and patient
- Unwanted effects of medical and surgical treatments
- History of mood disorder or misuse of alcohol or drugs
- Personality traits hindering adjustment, such as rigidity, pessimism, extreme need for independence and control
- Concurrent life events or social difficulties
- Lack of support from family and friends

Common causes of organic mental disorders

- Prescribed drugs—opioids, psychotropic drugs, corticosteroids, some cytotoxic drugs
- Infection—respiratory or urinary infection, septicaemia
- Macroscopic brain pathology—primary or secondary tumour, Alzheimer's disease, cerebrovascular disease, HIV dementia
- Metabolic—dehydration, electrolyte disturbance, hypercalcaemia, organ failure
- Drug withdrawal—benzodiazepines, opioids, alcohol

Confusion

This may present as forgetfulness, disorientation in time and place, and changes in mood or behaviour. The two main clinical syndromes are dementia (chronic brain syndrome), which is usually permanent, and delirium (acute brain syndrome), which is potentially reversible.

Delirium, which is more relevant to palliative care, comprises clouding of consciousness with various other abnormalities of mental function from an organic cause. Severity often fluctuates, worsening at night. Dehydration, neglect of personal hygiene, and accidental self injury may hasten physical and mental decline. Noisy, demanding, or aggressive behaviour may upset or harm other people. So called "terminal anguish" is a combination of delirium and overwhelming anxiety in the last few days of life. A physical cause usually contributes to "terminal anguish."

Recognition

Various misconceptions about psychiatric disorders in medical patients contribute to their widespread under-recognition and undertreatment. Education and training in communication skills, for both patients and staff, could help to remedy this.

Standardised screening instruments that have been validated for use in palliative care patients include the Edinburgh depression scale and the minimental state (MMS) or mental status schedule (MSS) for cognitive impairment. Though not sensitive or specific enough to substitute for assessment by interview, they can help to detect unsuspected cases, contribute to diagnostic assessment of probable cases, and provide a baseline for monitoring progress.

Knowledge of previous personality and psychological state is helpful in identifying high risk patients or those with evolving symptoms, and relatives' observations of any recent change should be obtained.

Prevention and management

General guidelines for both prevention and management include providing an explanation about the illness in the context of ongoing supportive relationships with known and trusted professionals. Patients should have the opportunity to express their feelings without fear of censure or abandonment. This facilitates the process of adjustment, helping patients to move on towards accepting their situation and making the most of their remaining life.

Visits from a specialist palliative care nurse or attendance at a palliative care day centre, combined with follow-up by the primary healthcare team, often benefit both patients and families. An opportunity to explore and express spiritual concerns is often helpful for all those patients, including those with no specific religious belief. Psychiatric referral is indicated when emotional disturbances are severe, atypical, or resistant to treatment; when there is concern about suicide; and on the rare occasions when compulsory measures under the Mental Health Act 1983 seem to be indicated.

Non-pharmacological therapies increase a patient's sense of participation and control. Usually delivered in regular planned sessions, they can also help in acute situations—for example, deep breathing, relaxation techniques, or massage for acute anxiety or panic attacks.

Symptoms and signs of depression

Somatic
- Reduced energy, fatigue
- Disturbed sleep, especially early morning waking
- Diminished appetite
- Psychomotor agitation or retardation

Psychological
- Low mood present most of the time, characteristically worse in the morning
- Loss of interest and pleasure
- Reduced concentration and attention
- Indecisiveness
- Feelings of guilt or worthlessness
- Pessimistic or hopeless ideas about the future
- Suicidal thoughts or acts

Symptoms and signs of anxiety

Psychological
- Apprehension, worry, inability to relax
- Difficulty in concentrating, irritability
- Difficulty falling asleep, unrefreshing sleep, nightmares

Motor tension
- Muscular aches and fatigue
- Restlessness, trembling, jumpiness
- Tension headaches

Autonomic
- Shortness of breath, palpitations, lightheadedness, dizziness
- Sweating, dry mouth, "lump in throat"
- Nausea, diarrhoea, urinary frequency

Symptoms and signs of delirium
- Clouding of consciousness (reduced awareness of environment)
- Impaired attention
- Impaired memory, especially recent memory
- Impaired abstract thinking and comprehension
- Disorientation in time, place, or person
- Perceptual distortions—illusions and hallucinations, usually visual or tactile
- Transient delusions, usually paranoid
- Psychomotor disturbance—agitation or underactivity
- Disturbed cycle of sleeping and waking, nightmares
- Emotional disturbance—depression, anxiety, fear, irritability, euphoria, apathy, perplexity

---

Why psychiatric disorders go unrecognised
- Patients are reluctant to voice emotional complaints—fear of seeming weak or ungrateful; stigma
- Professionals are reluctant to inquire—lack of time, lack of skill, emotional self protection
- Attributing somatic symptoms to medical illness
- Assuming emotional distress is inevitable and untreatable

For bedridden patients who are anxious or confused as well as sick, it is important to provide nursing care from a few trusted people; a quiet, familiar, safe, and comfortable environment; explanation of any practical procedure in advance; and an opportunity to discuss underlying fears.

The relatives' need for explanation and support must not be forgotten.

Psychotropic drugs

For more severe cases, drug treatment is indicated in addition to, not instead of, the general measures described above.

Depression

Drugs should be prescribed if a definite depressive syndrome is present or if a depressive adjustment reaction fails to resolve within a few weeks. The antidepressant effect of all these drugs takes at least four to six weeks to become evident.

Tricyclic antidepressants produce a worthwhile response in about 80% of patients but have considerable anticholinergic side effects in the doses necessary for a therapeutic response and therefore are not routinely indicated in palliative care settings.

Selective serotonin reuptake inhibitors such as sertraline (50 mg daily) or paroxetine (20 mg daily) have few anticholinergic effects, are non-sedative, and are safe in overdose. They may, however, cause nausea, diarrhoea, headache, or anxiety. The newer antidepressants, such as mirtazapine, seem to be better tolerated.

Other treatments—The use of drugs such as lithium or combinations of antidepressants should be prescribed and managed in consultation with a psychiatrist. Psychostimulants can be used but care needs to be taken regarding doses.

Anxiety

Benzodiazepines are best limited to short term or intermittent use; prolonged use may lead to a decline in anxiolytic effect and cumulative psychomotor impairment. Low dose neuroleptic drugs such as haloperidol 1.5–5 mg daily are an alternative. β blockers are useful for autonomic overactivity. Chronic anxiety is often better treated with a course of antidepressant drugs, especially if depression coexists.

Acute severe anxiety can present as an emergency. It may mask a medical problem—such as pain, pulmonary embolism, internal haemorrhage, or drug or alcohol withdrawal—or it may have been provoked by psychological trauma such as seeing another patient die. Whether or not the underlying cause is amenable to specific treatment, sedation is usually required. Lorazepam, a short acting benzodiazepine, can be given as 1 mg or 2.5 mg tablets orally or sublingually. Alternatively, midazolam 5–10 mg can be given subcutaneously. An antipsychotic such as haloperidol 5–10 mg may be more appropriate if the patient is also psychotic or confused. Medical assessment needs to be repeated every few hours, and the continued presence of a skilled and sympathetic companion is helpful.

Confusion

It is best to identify any treatable medical causes before prescribing further drugs, which may make the confusion worse. In practice, however, sedation maybe required. For mild nocturnal confusion, an antipsychotic such as haloperidol 1.5–5 mg at bedtime is often sufficient. For severe delirium, a single dose of haloperidol 5–10 mg may be offered in tablet or liquid form and a benzodiazepine can be added.

It may be possible to withdraw the drugs after one or two days if reversible factors such as infection or dehydration have

Principles of psychological management
- Sensitive breaking of bad news
- Providing information in accord with individual wishes
- Permitting expression of emotion
- Clarification of concerns and problems
- Patient involved in making decisions about treatment
- Setting realistic goals
- Appropriate package of medical, psychological, and social care
- Continuity of care from named staff

Some psychological and practical therapies
- Brief psychotherapy—cognitive-behavioural, cognitive-analytic, problem solving
- Group discussions for information and support
- Music therapy
- Art therapy
- Creative writing
- Relaxation techniques
- Meditation
- Hypnotherapy
- Aromatherapy
- Practical activity—such as craft work, swimming

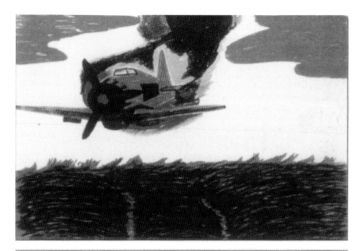

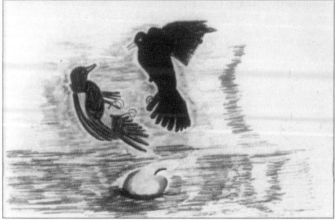

Examples of art therapy—the painter of these figures is a man with cancer of the larynx. Having lost his voice, his partner, and his hobby of playing the trumpet, he was depressed, angry, and in pain. He likened himself to an aircraft being shot down in flames or to a frightened bird at the mercy of a larger bird of prey. He has since improved and wrote to tell his doctor how much it helped to draw his "awful thoughts" (with permission from Camilla Connell, art therapist at Royal Marsden Hospital)

been dealt with. Otherwise, sedation may need to be continued until death, preferably by continuous subcutaneous infusion, for which a suitable regimen might be as much as haloperidol 10–30 mg with midazolam 30–60 mg every 24 hours. These drugs can be mixed in the same syringe.

Outcome

It is vitally important to be as vigilant for symptoms of anxiety, depression, and confusion in these patients as it is for physical symptoms. Symptoms such as anxiety or depression should never be considered inevitable. Prompt assessment of such symptoms together with appropriate management can greatly improve the overall quality of life for all patients.

Further reading
- Barraclough J. *Cancer and emotion*. Chichester: John Wiley, 1994.
- Lloyd-Williams M, ed. *Psychosocial issues in palliative care*. Oxford: Oxford University Press, 2003.

10 Emergencies

Stephen Falk, Colette Reid

Emergencies in most medical specialties are immediate life threatening events and successful outcome is measured by prolongation of life. While prolongation of life is rarely the main goal in palliative care, some acute events have to be treated as an emergency if a favourable outcome is to be achieved. As in any emergency, the assessment must be as prompt and complete as possible. In patients with advanced malignancy, factors to consider include:

- The nature of the emergency
- The general physical condition of the patient
- Disease status and likely prognosis
- Concomitant pathologies
- Symptoms
- The likely effectiveness and toxicity of available treatments
- Wishes of patient and carers.

While unnecessary hospital admission may cause distress for the patient and carers, missed emergency treatment of reversible symptoms can be disastrous.

Hypercalcaemia

Hypercalcaemia is the most common life threatening metabolic disorder encountered in patients with cancer. The incidence varies with the underlying malignancy, being most common in multiple myeloma and breast cancer (40–50%), less so in non-small cell lung cancer, and rare in small cell lung cancer and colorectal cancer.

It is important to remember the existence of non-malignant causes of hypercalcaemia—particularly primary hyperparathyroidism, which is prevalent in the general population.

The pathology of hypercalcaemia is mediated by factors such as parathyroid related protein, prostaglandins, and local interaction by cytokines such as interleukin 1 and tumour necrosis factor. Bone metastases are commonly but not invariably present.

Management

Mild hypercalcaemia (corrected serum calcium concentration ≤3.00 mmol/1) is usually asymptomatic, and treatment is required only if a patient has symptoms. For more severe hypercalcaemia, however, treatment can markedly improve symptoms even when a patient has advanced disease and limited life expectancy to make the end stages less traumatic for the patient and carers.

Treatment with bisphosphonate normalises the serum calcium concentration in 80% of patients within a week. Treatment with calcitonin or mithramycin is now largely obsolete. Corticosteroids are probably useful only when the underlying tumour is responsive to this cytostatic agent—such as myeloma, lymphoma, and some carcinomas of the breast.

Some symptoms, particularly confusion, may be slow to improve after treatment, despite normalisation of the serum calcium concentration. Always consider treating the underlying malignancy to prevent recurrence of symptoms as the median duration of normocalcaemia after bisphosphonate infusion is only three weeks. If effective systemic therapy has been exhausted, or is deemed inappropriate, however, oral bisphosphonates (such as clodronate 800 mg twice daily) or parenteral infusions (every three to four weeks) should be considered.

Maintenance intravenous bisphosphonates may be administered at a day centre or outpatient department. Oral preparations have the disadvantages of being poorly absorbed and have to be taken at least an hour before or after food. A recent systematic review suggests there is more evidence to support the intravenous route.

Obstruction of superior vena cava

This may arise from occlusion by extrinsic pressure, intraluminal thrombosis, or direct invasion of the vessel wall. Most cases are due to tumour within the mediastinum, of which up to 75% will be primary bronchial carcinomas. About 3% of patients with carcinoma of the bronchus and 8% of those with lymphoma will develop obstruction.

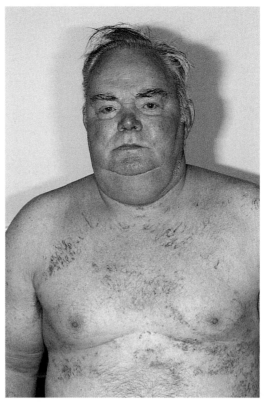

Patient with superior vena caval obstruction showing typical signs (reproduced with patient's permission)

Aetiology of obstruction of superior vena cava

Carcinoma of the bronchus	65–80%
Lymphoma	2–10%
Other cancers	3–13%
Benign causes (now rare)	Benign goiter, aortic aneurysm (syphilis), thrombotic syndromes, idiopathic sclerosing mediastinitis
Unknown or undiagnosed	5%

Management

Conventionally, obstruction of the superior vena cava has been regarded as an oncological emergency requiring immediate treatment. If it is the first presentation of malignancy, treatment will be tempered by the need to obtain an accurate histological diagnosis to tailor treatment for potentially curable diseases, such as lymphomas or germ cell tumours, and for diseases such as small cell lung cancer that are better treated with chemotherapy at presentation.

In advanced disease, patients need relief from acute symptoms—of which dyspnoea and a sensation of drowning can be most frightening—and high dose corticosteroids and radiotherapy or chemotherapy should be considered. In non-small cell lung cancer palliative radiotherapy gives symptomatic improvement in 60% of patients, with a median duration of palliation of three months. Up to 17% of patients may survive for a year. If radiotherapy is contraindicated or being awaited, corticosteroids alone (dexamethasone 16 mg/day) may give relief. Stenting (with or without thrombolysis) of the superior vena cava should be considered for both small cell and non-small cell lung cancer either as initial treatment or for relapse.

Urgent initiation of pharmacological, practical, and psychological management of dyspnoea is paramount and usually includes opioids, with or without benzodiazepines. Opioid doses are usually small—such as 5 mg oral morphine every four hours. It is important to review all prescriptions of corticosteroids in view of their potential adverse effects. We recommend stopping corticosteroids after five days if no benefit is obtained and a gradual reduction in dose for those who have responded.

Clinical features of superior vena caval obstruction

Symptoms
- Tracheal oedema and shortness of breath
- Cerebral oedema with headache worse on stooping
- Visual changes
- Dizziness and syncope
- Swelling of face, particularly periorbital oedema
- Neck swelling
- Oedema of arms and hands

Clinical signs
- Rapid breathing
- Periorbital oedema
- Suffused injected conjunctivae
- Cyanosis
- Non-pulsatile distension of neck veins
- Dilated collateral superficial veins of upper chest
- Oedema of hands and arms

Spinal cord compression

Compression of the spinal cord occurs in up to 5% of patients with cancer. The main problem in clinical practice is failure of recognition. It is not uncommon for a patient's weak legs to be attributed to general debility and urinary and bowel symptoms to be attributed to medication. Neurological symptoms and signs can vary from subtle to gross, from upper motor neurone

Presentation of spinal cord compression can be subtle in the early stages. Any patient with back pain and subtle neurological symptoms or signs should have radiological investigations, with magnetic resonance imaging when possible

to lower motor neurone, and from minor sensory changes to clearly demarcated sensory loss.

Prompt treatment is essential if function is to be maintained: neurological status at the start of treatment is the most important factor to influence outcome. If treatment is started within 24–48 hours of onset of symptoms neurological damage may be reversible.

Reasons for delay in treatment of spinal cord compression

- Failure to recognise from early symptoms
- Lack of clear referral pathway
- No investigation pathway

Spinal cord compression can arise from intradural metastasis but is more commonly extradural in origin. In 85% of cases cord damage arises from extension of a vertebral body metastasis into the epidural space, but other mechanisms of damage include vertebral collapse, direct spread of tumour through the intervertebral foramen (usually in lymphoma or testicular tumour), and interruption of the vascular supply.

The frequency with which a particular spinal level is affected reflects the number and volume of vertebral bodies in each segment—about 10% of compressions are cervical, 70% thoracic, and 20% lumbosacral. It is important to remember that more than one site of compression may occur, and this is increasingly recognised with improved imaging techniques. Decisions on investigations performed and treatment given will depend on the patient's wishes and the stage of the disease. Only in exceptional circumstances will corticosteroids not form part of the treatment plan.

The earliest symptom of spinal cord compression is back pain, sometimes with symptoms of root irritation, causing a girdle-like pain, which is often described as a "band" that tends to be worse on coughing or straining. Most patients have pain for weeks or months before they start to detect weakness. Initially, stiffness rather than weakness may be a feature, and tingling and numbness usually starts in both feet and ascends the legs. In contrast with pain, the start of myelopathy is usually rapid. Urinary symptoms such as hesitancy or incontinence and perianal numbness are late features. Increasing compression of the spinal cord is often marked by improvement or resolution of the back pain but can be associated with worsening of pain.

Examination may reveal a defined area of sensory loss and brisk or absent reflexes, which may help to localise the lesion. In patients unfit to undergo more detailed investigations, plain radiology can reveal erosion of the pedicles, vertebral collapse, and, occasionally, a large paravertebral mass. These may help in the application of palliative radiotherapy. In contrast with myelography with localised computed tomographic x-rays for soft tissue detail, magnetic resonance imaging is now considered the investigation of choice: it is non-invasive and shows the whole spine, enabling detection of multiple areas of compression.

Management

After palliative radiotherapy, 70% of patients who were ambulatory at the start of treatment retain their ability to walk and 35% of patients with paraparesis regain their ability to walk, while only 5% of completely paraplegic patients do so. These figures underline the importance of early diagnosis, as 75% of patients have substantial weakness at presentation to oncology units.

Retrospective analysis has not shown an advantage for patients managed by laminectomy and radiotherapy over radiotherapy alone. A recent prospective study, however, has

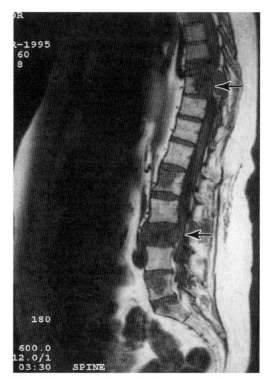

Magnetic resonance image showing patient with spinal cord compression at two different sites (arrows)

Management of spinal cord compression

Main points
- Except for unusual circumstances give oral dexamethasone 16 mg/day
- Urgent treatment, definitely within 24 hours of start of symptoms
- Interdisciplinary approach involving oncologists, neurosurgeons, radiologists, nurses, physiotherapists, occupational therapists

Treatment options
- Continue with dexamethasone 16 mg/day *plus*
- Radiation only
  For most situations
  Radiosensitive tumour without spinal instability
- Surgery and radiation
  Spinal instability, such as fracture or compression by bone
  No tissue diagnosis (when needle biopsy guided by computed tomography is not possible)
- Surgery only
  Relapse at previously irradiated area
  Progression during radiotherapy
- Chemotherapy
  Paediatric tumours responsive to chemotherapy
  Adjuvant treatment for adult tumours responsive to chemotherapy
  Relapse of previously irradiated tumour responsive to chemotherapy
- Corticosteroids alone
  Final stages of terminal illness and patient either too unwell to have radiotherapy or unlikely to live long enough to receive any benefits

---

indicated that radiotherapy plus surgery obtained more functional benefit than radiotherapy alone, even in those patients with initial poor performance status.

Surgical decompression is also indicated for cases when:

- A tissue diagnosis is required (if biopsy guided by computed tomography is not possible)
- Deterioration occurs during radiotherapy
- There is bone destruction causing spinal cord compression.

For a small number of fit patients with disease anterior to the spinal canal, excellent results have been reported for an anterior approach for surgical decompression and vertebral stabilisation—80% of the patients became ambulant. For relief of the mechanical problems due to bone collapse, laminectomy decompression has to be accompanied by spinal stabilisation. Such surgery is difficult and not always appropriate.

Bone fracture

Bone metastases are a common feature of advanced cancer. Bone fracture may also be due to osteoporosis or trauma. Fractures can present in various forms, including as an acute confusional state.

Management
If fracture of a long bone seems likely, as judged by the presence of cortical thinning, prophylactic internal fixation should be considered. Once a fracture has occurred the available options include external or internal fixation; the site of the fracture and the general condition of the patient determines their relative merits.

Radiotherapy is usually given in an attempt to enhance healing and to prevent further progression of the bony metastasis and subsequent loosening of any fixation.

Evidence exists that, when combined with oncolytic therapy in most solid tumours, oral bisphosphonates can reduce skeletal morbidity (hypercalcaemia, vertebral fracture, and need for palliative radiotherapy).

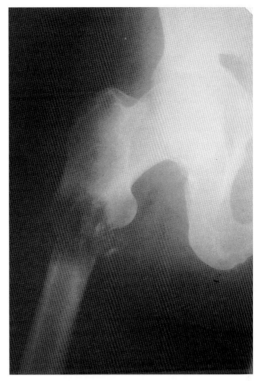

Radiograph showing pathological fracture of the femur

Further reading
- Doyle D, Hanks G, Cherny N, Calman, K, eds. *Oxford textbook of palliative medicine*. 3rd ed. Oxford: Oxford University Press, 2003.
- Levack P, Graham J, Collie D, Grant R, Kidd J, Kunkler I, et al. Don't wait for a sensory level—listen to the symptoms: a prospective audit of the delays in diagnosis of malignant cord compression. *Clin Oncol (R Coll Radiol)* 2002;14:472–80.
- Ross JR, Saunders Y, Edmonds PM, Patel S, Broadley KE, Johnston SRD. Systematic review of role of bisphosphonates on skeletal morbidity in metastatic cancer. *BMJ* 2003;327:469–74.
- Rowell NP, Gleeson FV. Steroids, radiotherapy, chemotherapy and stents for superior vena caval obstruction in carcinoma of the bronchus. *Cochrane Database Syst Rev* 2005;(2):CD001316.

11 The last 48 hours

James Adam

During the last 48 hours of life, patients experience increasing weakness and immobility, loss of interest in food and drink, difficulty in swallowing, and drowsiness. Signs may include a new gauntness, changes in breathing pattern, cool and sometimes oedematous peripheries, and cognitive impairment. With an incurable and progressive illness, this phase can usually be anticipated, but sometimes the deterioration can be sudden and distressing. Control of the symptoms and support of the family take priority, and the nature of the primary illness becomes less important. This is a time when levels of anxiety, stress, and emotion can be high for patients, families, and other carers. It is important that the healthcare team adopts a sensitive yet structured approach.

The Liverpool care pathway (LCP)
This pathway provides multidisciplinary documentation and prompted guidelines towards achieving important goals for patients with cancer and their families in the dying phase. Although it was developed in a hospice, there are adaptations for acute and community settings that encourage discussion around the diagnosis of dying and reduction of unnecessary or futile interventions (including CPR) at this stage. It also provides a means to measure symptom control in the dying patient and, through analysis of variance, identify educational and resource needs.

Identifying when death seems imminent
(from the Liverpool care pathway)

The multiprofessional team has agreed that the patient is dying, and two of the following may apply:
- Bed bound
- Semicomatose
- Only able to take sips of fluid
- No longer able to take tablets

Principles

An analytical approach to symptom control continues but usually relies on clinical findings rather than investigation. This approach spans all causes of terminal illness and applies to care at home, hospital, or hospice.

Drugs are reviewed with regard to need and route of administration. Previously "essential" drugs such as antihypertensives, corticosteroids, antidepressants, and hypoglycaemics are often no longer needed and analgesic, antiemetic, sedative, and anticonvulsant drugs form the new "essential" list to work from. The route of administration depends on the clinical situation and characteristics of the drugs used. Some patients manage to take oral drugs until near to death, but many require an alternative route. Any change in medication relies on information from the patient, family, and carers (both lay and professional) and regular medical review to monitor the level of symptom control and side effects.

This review should include an assessment of how the family and carers are coping; effective communication with all involved should be maintained and lines of communication made clear and open and documented if appropriate. The knowledge that help is available is often a reassurance and can influence the place of death.

Principles of managing the last 48 hours
- Problem solving approach to symptom control
- Avoid unnecessary interventions
- Review all drugs and symptoms regularly
- Maintain effective communication
- Ensure support for family and carers

Routes of administration for drugs used in last 48 hours

Route	Drug
Oral	
All drug types	
Sublingual	
Antiemetic	Hyoscine hydrobromide 0.3 mg/6 hours (Kwells)
Sedative or anxiolytic	Lorazepam 0.5–2.5 mg/6 hours (fast acting)
Transdermal	
Opioid	Fentanyl or buprenorphine (only if patient already on patches)
Antiemetic (Scopaderm)	Hyoscine hydrobromide 1 mg/72 hours
Subcutaneous*	
Opioids	Diamorphine (individual dose titration) Oxycodone and alfentanil may be alternatives where there is morphine intolerance
NSAIDs	Diclofenac (infusion) 150 mg/24 hours
Antiemetics	Cyclizine 25–50 mg/8 hours: up to 150 mg/24 hours
	Metoclopramide 10 mg/6 hours: 40–80 mg/24 hours
	Levomepromazine 6.25–25 mg bolus: 6.25 mg titrated up to 250 mg/24 hours via syringe driver (sedating at higher doses)
	Haloperidol (also useful for confusion with altered sensorium associated with opioid toxicity) 2.5–5 mg bolus: 5–30 mg/24 hours
Sedative, anxiolytic, anticonvulsant	Midazolam 2.5–10 mg bolus: 5–60 mg/24 hours (anticonvulsant starting dose 30 mg/24 hours)
	Phenobarbitone (for refractory cases)
Antisecretory	Hyoscine hydrobromide 0.4–0.6 mg bolus; 2.4 mg/24 hours
	Glycopyrronium and hyoscine butylbromide (non-sedating alternatives)
Somatostatin analogue	Octreotide (for large volume vomit associated with bowel obstruction) 300–600 µg/24 hours
Rectal	
Opioids	Morphine 15–30 mg/4 hours Oxycodone 30–60 mg/8 hours (named patient only)
NSAIDs	Diclofenac 100 mg once daily
Antiemetic	Domperidone 30–60 mg/6 hours Prochlorperazine 25 mg twice daily Cyclizine 50 mg three times a day
Sedative and anxiolytic	Diazepam rectal tubes (also anticonvulsant) 5–10 mg/2.5 ml tubes

*All preparations diluted in sterile water except diclofenac (0.9% saline)

Symptom control

Pain

Pain control is achievable in 80% of patients by following the WHO guidelines for use of analgesic drugs, as outlined in chapter 2. A patient's history and examination are used to assess all likely causes of pain, both benign and malignant. Treatment (usually with an opioid) is individually tailored, the effect reviewed, and doses titrated accordingly. Acute episodes of pain are dealt with urgently in the same analytical fashion but require more frequent review and provision of appropriate "breakthrough" analgesia. If a patient is already receiving analgesia then this is continued through the final stages; pain may disturb an unconscious patient as the original cause of the pain still exists.

If oral administration is no longer possible the subcutaneous route provides a simple and effective alternative. Diamorphine is the strong opioid of choice because of its solubility and is delivered through an infusion device to avoid repeated injections every four hours. It can be mixed with other "essential" drugs in the syringe driver. Oxycodone and alfentanil can be infused subcutaneously in cases of genuine morphine intolerance. Rectal administration is another alternative, but the need for suppositories every four hours in the case of morphine limits its usefulness. Oxycodone suppositories (repeated every eight hours) may be more practicable.

Longer acting opioid preparations (transdermal fentanyl and sustained release opioids) should not be started in a patient close to death; there is a variable delay in reaching effective levels, and, as speedy dose titration is difficult, they are unsuitable for situations where a rapid effect is required, such as uncontrolled pain. If a patient is already prescribed fentanyl patches these should be continued as baseline analgesia; if pain escalates additional quick acting analgesia (immediate release morphine or diamorphine) should be titrated against the pain with appropriate breakthrough doses.

Not all pains are best dealt with by opioids. For example, a non-steroidal anti-inflammatory drug may help in bone pain, while muscle spasm may be eased by diazepam. It is also important to remember all the non-cancer pains, new and old, that may be present.

Breathlessness

The scope for correcting "reversible" causes of breathlessness becomes limited. A notable exception is cardiac failure, for which diuresis may be effective. In most cases the priority is to address the symptom of breathlessness and the fear and anxiety that may accompany it.

General supportive measures should be considered in all cases. Face masks may be uncomfortable or intrusive at this time, but oxygen therapy may help some patients (even in the absence of hypoxia) who are breathless at rest. Nebulised 0.9% saline is useful if a patient has a dry cough or sticky secretions but should be avoided if bronchospasm is present.

Opioids and benzodiazepines can be helpful and should be initiated at low doses. Immediate release morphine can be titrated to effect in the same way as for pain. If a patient is using morphine for pain control then a dose slightly higher than the appropriate breakthrough dose (oral or parenteral) is usually required for treating acute breathlessness. The choice of anxiolytic is often determined by what is the most suitable route of administration, but the speed and duration of action are also important.

Opioid treatment for pain control

- *Starting dose*—Immediate release morphine 5 mg every four hours by mouth
- *Increments*—A third of current dose (but varies according to "breakthrough analgesia" required in previous 24 hours). For example, immediate release morphine 15 mg every four hours by mouth is increased to 20 mg every four hours
- *Breakthrough analgesia*—A sixth of 24 hour dose. For example, with diamorphine 60 mg delivered subcutaneously by syringe driver over 24 hours, give diamorphine 10 mg subcutaneously as needed for breakthrough pain
- *Conversion ratio*—Morphine by mouth (or rectum) to subcutaneous diamorphine is 3:1. For example, sustained release morphine 30 mg every 12 hours by mouth plus three doses of immediate release morphine 10 mg by mouth gives total dose of oral morphine 90 mg every 24 hours; convert to diamorphine 30 mg/24 hours delivered subcutaneously

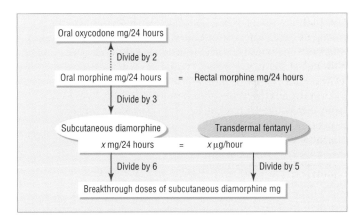

A guide to equivalent doses and appropriate breakthrough doses in opioid analgesics

Non-drug measures for pain

Type of pain	Measure
Dry mouth	Mouth care
Pressure sore	Change of position
	Comfort dressing
	Local anaesthetic gel
	Appropriate mattress
Distended bladder	Catheterisation
Loaded rectum	Rectal evacuation

Management of breathlessness

- Reverse what is reversible
- General supportive measures—explanation, position, breathing exercises, fan or cool airflow, relaxation techniques
- Oxygen therapy
- Opioid
- Benzodiazepine
- Hyoscine
- Nebulised saline (if there is no bronchospasm and the patient is able to expectorate)

Noisy respiration may be helped by repositioning the patient and, if substantial secretions are present, use of hyoscine hydrobromide (0.4–0.6 mg subcutaneous bolus or up to 2.4 mg/24 hours via infusion device). Hyoscine butylbromide (20 mg subcutaneous bolus; up to 120 mg/24 hrs) and glycopyrronium (0.4 mg subcutaneous bolus; up to 1.2 mg/24 hrs) are non-sedating alternatives. Occasionally, gentle suction may be required. End stage stridor is managed with opioids and anxiolytics, as it is usually too late for corticosteroids.

Restlessness and confusion

These may be distinct entities or they may overlap. A problem solving approach is essential. The threshold for discomfort and disorientation is often lowered in cachectic or anxious patients. Attention to a patient's surroundings is therefore important—a stable, comfortable, and safe environment should be fostered; soft light, quiet, explanation, and familiar faces are reassuring.

The key to treatment lies in calming the acute state while dealing with the cause, if it is apparent and appropriate. A notable example is the mental clouding, hallucinations, confusion, and restlessness associated with opioid toxicity, which can be eased with haloperidol while the opioid dose is reviewed. In general, choice of drug treatment depends on the likely cause. Doses are titrated up or down to achieve the desired effect, and the situation should be reviewed regularly and often until the acute episode settles. Highly agitated patients may need a large dose, and continuous infusion may be needed. Rectally administered drugs are possible alternatives. Explanation and support for the relatives and carers are paramount at this time.

If a patient is experiencing distressing twitching or jerks then major organ failure and metabolic disorders are possible, but opioid toxicity, drugs that lower seizure threshold, and withdrawal of anticonvulsants should be considered. A review of medication and treatment with a benzodiazepine or anticonvulsant (such as clonazepam orally, diazepam rectally, or midazolam subcutaneously) is indicated. Anxiety or distress that does not respond to general supportive measures may be helped by diazepam or midazolam, but it should always be remembered that a patient may be suffering from emotional or spiritual anguish that cannot be relieved by drugs.

Nausea and vomiting

If antiemetics have been needed within the previous 24 hours then continuation is advisable. Nausea and vomiting may rarely occur as a new symptom at this time (<10% of cases), and treatment of the likely cause is preferred if this is practical in the clinical situation, otherwise an appropriate antiemetic should be selected. If the aetiology is unclear then choose a centrally acting or broad spectrum antiemetic in the first instance.

Occasionally, more than one antiemetic is required if resistant vomiting of a multifactorial cause exists. Subcutaneous administration of antiemetics is preferable, but suppositories (such as prochlorperazine, cyclizine, or domperidone) may be useful if subcutaneous infusion is not possible. Antiemetic treatment that has been initiated for bowel obstruction should be continued.

Emergency situations

Appropriate and timely action has an important immediate effect on patients and families. It can also influence bereavement and future coping mechanisms of both lay and professional carers. Emergencies can sometimes be anticipated: previous haemoptysis may predict haemorrhage, bone

---

Causes of restlessness and confusion

- Drugs—such as opioids, corticosteroids, neuroleptics, alcohol (intoxication and withdrawal)
- Physical—unrelieved pain, distended bladder or bowel, immobility or exhaustion, cerebral lesions, infection, haematological abnormalities, major organ failure
- Metabolic upset—urea, calcium, sodium, glucose, hypoxia
- Anxiety and distress

Management of restlessness and confusion

- Treat the acute state and deal with the cause
- General supportive measures—light, reassurance, company
- Choice of drug treatment relates to likely cause

Drugs
- Haloperidol
  Indications—Drug toxicity, altered sensorium, metabolic upset
  Dose—Oral drug 1.5–3 mg, repeat after one hour and review; subcutaneous bolus 2.5–10 mg; subcutaneous infusion 5–30 mg over 24 hours
- Midazolam
  Indications—Anxiety and distress, risk of seizure
  Dose—Subcutaneous bolus 2.5–10 mg; subcutaneous infusion 5–100 mg over 24 hours
- Levomepromazine
  Indications—Need for alternative or additional sedation
  Dose—Subcutaneous bolus 25 mg; subcutaneous infusion up to 250 mg over 24 hours (lowers seizure threshold, use with care)
- For altered sensorium plus anxiety, combine haloperidol and midazolam
- Avoid "slippery slope" of inappropriate sedation in patient who needs to talk; so called "terminal agitation" can result from the inappropriate use of drugs

---

Causes and treatment of nausea and vomiting

Site of effect	Treatment
Drugs or biochemical upset Chemoreceptor trigger zone (area postrema) via dopamine receptors	Haloperidol
Raised intracranial pressure Vomiting centre via histamine receptors	Cyclizine
Multifactorial or uncertain aetiology Various	Levomepromazine
Gastrointestinal stasis Gastrokinetic	Metoclopramide
Bowel obstruction Vomiting centre via vagus nerve Gastrointestinal secretions	Cyclizine (or levomepromazine) Octreotide (or hyoscine) butylbromide

metastases predict pathological fracture, enlarging upper airway tumour predicts stridor, and previous hypercalcaemia predict confusion.

Some emergencies may be preventable. For example, a patient with a brain tumour who can no longer take corticosteroids with or without an anticonvulsant may have a seizure unless anticonvulsant treatment is maintained: subcutaneous infusion of midazolam (starting at 30 mg/24 hours) and rectally administered diazepam (10 mg) may be the strategy required. Phenobarbitone may be useful in refractory cases.

Most emergencies in the last 48 hours, however, are irreversible, and treatment should be aimed at the urgent relief of distress and concomitant symptoms. Drugs should be made available for immediate administration by nursing staff without further consultation with a doctor. Directions regarding use should be written clearly in unambiguous language. Useful drugs are injections of midazolam (5–10 mg if the patient has no previous exposure to benzodiazepine, otherwise titrate as appropriate) and diamorphine (5–10 mg if no previous exposure to opioid, otherwise a sixth to a third of the 24 hour dose).

Haemorrhage is distressing and unforgettable for both patients and carers. Haemoptysis, haematemesis, and erosion of a major artery such as the carotid are visually traumatic. The prompt use of drugs, dark coloured towels to make the view less distressing (green surgical towels in hospital), and warmth will aid comfort. In these situations death may occur quickly. A supportive presence is helpful, and explanations to patients and their carers of what is being done will help to minimise distress in a crisis.

Support

Support means recognising and addressing the physical and emotional issues that may face patients, families, and carers during this time. Patients and carers value honesty, listening, availability, and assurance that symptom control will continue. Fears or religious concerns should be acknowledged and addressed appropriately, and respect for cultural differences should be assured. Explain what is happening, what is likely to happen, the drugs being used, the support available, and how the family can help with care.

Lack of practical support is one of the most common reasons for admission to hospital or hospice at this time, and, therefore, consideration should be given to extra help—such as Marie Curie nurses (organised through the district nursing service)—to give carers rest and support. An assessment of the risk of bereavement allows care to be planned for the family after the patient's death. Professional carers may also need support, particularly if the last 48 hours have been difficult, and this requires an open line of communication.

Emergencies
- Stridor
- Seizure
- Haemorrhage
- Pain
- Confusion

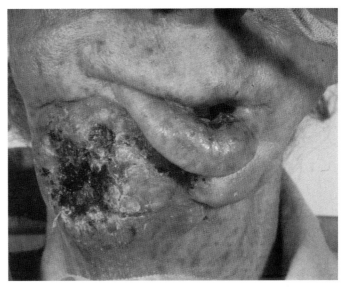

Patient with ulcerated neck tumour at risk of erosion of the carotid artery and massive bleed

Factors that can make bereavement more difficult
- Patient—young
- Illness—short, protracted, disfiguring, distressing
- Death—sudden, traumatic (such as haemorrhage)
- Relationship—ambivalent, hostile, dependent
- Main carer—young, other dependants, physical or mental illness, concurrent crises, little or no support

Further reading
- Doyle D, Hanks G, Cherney NI, Calman K, eds. *Oxford textbook of palliative medicine*. 3rd ed. Oxford: Oxford University Press, 2002.
- Ellershaw J, Wilkinson S, eds. *Care of the dying—a pathway to excellence*. Oxford: Oxford University Press, 2003.
- Twycross RG, Wilcock A, Charlesworth S, Dickman A. *Palliative care formulary*. 2nd ed. Abingdon, Oxon: Radcliffe Medical Press, 2002.

The table entitled "Identifying when death seems imminent" is reproduced with permission of Dr John Ellershaw.

12 Palliative care for children

Ann Goldman

The death of a child has long been acknowledged as one of the greatest tragedies that can happen to a family, and care for seriously ill children and their families is central to paediatrics. The needs for palliative care for children with life limiting illnesses and their families are now formally recognised within paediatrics in the UK. The most suitable approaches to care, however, are still evolving, and the training and provision of the necessary multidisciplinary workforce is being developed to provide a fully comprehensive national service in the UK.

In the US excellent research has provided us with a better understanding of management of symptoms, especially pain. Aspects of care vary greatly between countries but remain based with the attending physician.

Which children need care?

Fortunately, deaths in childhood that can be anticipated and for which palliative care can be planned are rare. A report by ACT (Association for Children with Life Threatening or Terminal Conditions and their Families) and the Royal College of Paediatrics and Child Health has recently been updated and offers the currently available information about epidemiology. It suggests that the number of children who would benefit from palliative care is higher than was previously thought.

Palliative care for children is offered for a wide range of life limiting conditions, which differ from adult diseases. Many of these are rare and familial. The diagnosis influences the type of care that a child and family will need, and four broad groups have been identified.

Palliative care may be needed from infancy and for many years for some children, while others may not need it until they are older and only for a short time. Also the transition from aggressive treatments aimed at curing the condition or prolonging good quality life to palliative care may not be clear. Both approaches may be needed in conjunction, each becoming dominant at different times.

Aspects of care in children

Child development
Childhood is a time of continuing physical, emotional, and cognitive development. This influences all aspects of the care of children, from pharmacodynamics and pharmacokinetics of drugs to the communication skills of the children and their understanding of their disease and death.

Care at home
Most children with a life limiting disease are cared for at home. Parents are at the same time part of the team caring for the sick child and part of the family, needing care themselves. As their child's primary carers, they must be included fully in the care team—provided with information, able to negotiate treatment plans, taught appropriate skills, and assured that advice and support is accessible 24 hours a day.

Assessing symptoms
Assessing symptoms is an essential step in developing a plan of management. Often a picture must be built up through discussion with the child, if possible, combined with careful observations by parents and staff. It is also important to

---

Groups of life limiting disease in children

Group	Examples
Diseases for which curative treatment may be feasible but may fail	Cancer
Diseases in which premature death is inevitable but where intensive treatment may prolong good quality life	Cystic fibrosis HIV/AIDS
Progressive diseases for which treatment is exclusively palliative and may extend over many years	Batten disease Mucopolysaccharidoses
Irreversible but non-progressive conditions leading to vulnerability and health complications likely to cause premature death	Severe cerebral palsy

---

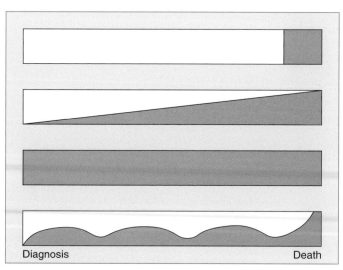

Palliative care (shaded) and treatments aiming to cure or prolong life (not shaded) vary in different situations and with time

---

Methods of assessing pain in children
- Body charts
- Faces scales
- Numeric scales
- Diaries
- Colour tools
- Visual analogue scales

consider the contribution of psychological and social factors for a child and family and to inquire about their coping strategies, relevant past experiences, and their levels of anxiety and emotional distress. There are formal assessment tools for assessing severity of pain in children that are appropriate for different ages and developmental levels, but assessment is more difficult for other symptoms and for preverbal and developmentally delayed children.

Managing symptoms
In all situations the management plan should consider both pharmacological and psychological approaches along with practical help.

Children often find it difficult to take large amounts of drugs, and complex regimens may not be possible. Doses should be calculated according to a child's weight. Oral drugs should be used if possible, and children should be offered the choice between tablets, whole or crushed, and liquids. Long acting transdermal and buccal preparations can be helpful, reducing the number of tablets needed and simplifying care at home. Some children find rectal drugs acceptable; they can be particularly useful in the last few days of life. Otherwise, a subcutaneous infusion can be established or, if one is in situ, a central intravenous line can be used. Parents are usually willing and able to learn to refill and load syringes and even to resite needles.

Specific problems

Pain
The myths perpetuating the undertreatment of pain in children have now been rejected. Most doctors, however, lack experience in using strong opioids in children, which often results in excessive caution. Also the difficulties of assessing pain, especially in preverbal and developmentally delayed children, can still result in lack of recognition and undertreatment of pain. After identifying the source of pain in a child appropriate analgesics and non-pharmacological approaches to pain management can be chosen. The WHO's three step ladder of analgesia is equally relevant for children, with paracetamol, codeine, and morphine forming the standard steps.

Opioids—Laxatives need to be prescribed regularly with opioids, but children rarely need antiemetics. With opioids, itching in the first few days is quite common and usually responds to antihistamines if necessary. Many children are sleepy initially, and parents should be warned of this lest they fear that their child's disease has suddenly progressed. Respiratory depression with strong opioids used in standard doses is not a problem in children over 1 year, but in younger children starting doses should be reduced.

Adjuvant analgesics—Non-steroidal anti-inflammatory drugs are often helpful for musculoskeletal pain in children with non-malignant disease. Caution is needed in children with cancer and infiltration of the bone marrow because of an increased risk of bleeding. Neuropathic pain may be helped by antiepileptic and antidepressant drugs. Pain from muscle spasms can be a major problem for children with neurodegenerative diseases and may be helped by benzodiazepines and baclofen.

Headaches from raised intracranial pressure associated with brain tumours are best managed with analgesic drugs used as described in the WHO guidelines. Although corticosteroids are often helpful initially, the symptoms soon recur and increasing doses are needed. The considerable side effects of corticosteroids in children—rapid weight gain, changed body image, and mood swings—usually outweigh the benefits. Headaches from leukaemic deposits in the central nervous

Paediatric pain profile
Items used by families and professionals in assessing pain in children with severe developmental delay. The child's own baseline levels are scored and compared with changes occurring with pain
- Was cheerful
- Was sociable or responsive
- Appeared withdrawn or depressed
- Cried/moaned/groaned/screamed or whimpered
- Was hard to console or comfort
- Self harmed—for example, bit self or banged head
- Was reluctant to eat/difficult to feed
- Had disturbed sleep
- Grimaced/screwed up face/screwed up eyes
- Frowned/had furrowed brow/looked worried
- Looked frightened (with eyes wide open)
- Ground teeth or made mouthing movements
- Was restless/agitated or distressed
- Tensed/stiffened or spasmed
- Flexed inwards or drew leg up towards chest
- Tended to touch or rub particular areas
- Resisted being moved
- Pulled away or flinched when touched
- Twisted and turned/tossed head/writhed or arched back
- Had involuntary or stereotypical movements/was jumpy/startled or had seizures

> Many of the drug doses and routes used in palliative care are not licensed for children, and this places an additional burden of responsibility with the clinician prescribing them

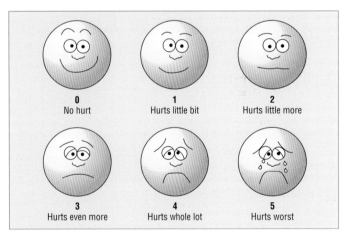

The Wong-Baker faces scale (adapted from Wong DL *et al.*, eds. *Whaley and Wong's essentials of pediatric nursing*. 5th ed. St Louis, MO: Mosby, 2001)

Children and pain
- Children's nervous systems do perceive pain
- Children do experience pain
- Children do remember pain
- Children are not more easily addicted to opioids
- There is no correct amount of pain or analgesia for a given injury

system respond well to intrathecal methotrexate.

Feeding

Being unable to nourish their child causes parents great distress and often makes them feel that they are failing as parents. Sucking and eating are part of children's development and provide comfort, pleasure, and stimulation. These aspects should be considered alongside a child's medical and practical problems with eating. Children with neurodegenerative disorders or brain tumours are particularly affected. In general, nutritional goals aimed at restoring health are secondary to comfort and enjoyment, although assisted feeding, via a nasogastric tube or gastrostomy, may be appropriate for those with slowly progressive disease.

Nausea and vomiting

These are common problems. Antiemetics can be selected according to their site of action and the presumed cause of the nausea (see chapter 7). In resistant cases combining a number of drugs that act in different ways can be helpful. Vomiting from raised intracranial pressure should be managed with cyclizine in the first instance.

Neurological problems

A grand mal fit in a child is extremely frightening for parents, and they should always be warned if it is a possibility and advised about management. A supply of buccal midazolam or rectal diazepam at home is valuable for managing seizures. Subcutaneous midazolam can enable parents to keep a child with severe repeated seizures at home. Maintenance antiepileptic medications for children with neurodegenerative disease may need adjusting as the illness progresses.

Agitation and anxiety may reflect a child's need to express his or her fears and distress. Drugs such as benzodiazepines, methotrimeprazine, and haloperidol may help to provide relief, especially in the final stages of life.

Support for the family

The needs of children and young people with a life threatening illness and their families are summarised in the report by ACT and the Royal College of Paediatrics and Child Health. Families need support from the time of diagnosis and throughout treatment, as well as when the disease is far advanced. Professionals must be flexible in their efforts to help. Each family and individual within a family is unique, with different strengths and coping skills. The needs of siblings and grandparents should be included. The family of a child with an inherited condition have additional difficulties. They may have feelings of guilt and blame, and they will need genetic counselling and information about prenatal diagnosis in the future. When an illness does not present until some years after birth, several children in the same family may be affected.

Families who maintain open communication cope most effectively, but this is not everyone's pattern. Children almost always know more than their parents think, and parents should be encouraged to be as honest as they can. Play material, books, and other resources can be supplied to help with communication, and parents can be helped to recognise their children's non-verbal cues.

Sick children need the opportunity to maintain their interests and to have short term goals for as long as possible. Play and education is an essential part of this, as they represent the normal pattern and help children to continue relationships with their peers. Providing information and support to teachers facilitates this.

Analgesic doses in children

Paracetamol
- Oral dose 15 mg/kg every four to six hours
- Rectal dose 20 mg/kg every six hours
- Maximum dose 90 mg/kg/24 hours; 60 mg/kg/24 hours in neonates

Dihydrocodeine
- Age <4 years 500 µg/kg orally every four to six hours
- Age 4–12 years 500–1000 µg/kg orally every four to six hours

Morphine
Immediate release preparations
- Age <1 year 150 µg/kg orally every four hours
- Age 1–12 years 200–400 µg/kg orally every four hours
- Age >12 years 10–15 mg orally every four hours
- Titrate according to analgesic effect and provide laxatives

12 hourly preparations
- Age <1 year 500 µg/kg orally every 12 hours
- Age 1–12 years 1 mg/kg orally every 12 hours
- Age >12 years 30 mg orally every 12 hours
- These are guidelines to starting doses, but many patients may start at higher doses after titration with immediate release morphine preparations every four hours

Diamorphine
- A third of total 24 hour doses of oral morphine
- Subcutaneous 24 hour infusion

Support that every child and family should expect

- To receive a flexible service according to a care plan based on individual assessment of needs, with reviews at appropriate intervals
- To have a named key worker to coordinate their care and provide access to appropriate professionals
- To be included in the caseload of a paediatrician in their home area and have access to local clinicians, nurses, and therapists skilled in children's palliative care and knowledgeable about services provided by agencies outside the NHS
- To be in the care of an identified lead consultant paediatrician expert in the individual child's condition
- To be supported in day to day management of child's physical and emotional symptoms and to have access to 24 hour care in the terminal stage
- To receive help in meeting the needs of parents and siblings, both during child's illness and during death and bereavement
- To be offered flexible respite and short term respite breaks including nursing care and symptom management both at home or in a children's hospice
- To be provided with drugs, oxygen, specialised feeds, and all disposable items such as feeding tubes, suction catheters, and stoma products through a single source
- To be provided with adaptations to housing and specialist equipment for use at home and school in an efficient and timely manner without recourse to several agencies
- To be helped in procuring benefits, grants, and other financial assistance

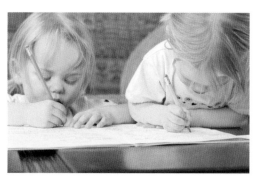

Play and education enable children to pursue short term goals (photos.com)

Bereavement

Grief after the death of a child is described as the most painful and enduring. Parents suffer multiple losses. Siblings suffer too and may have difficulty adjusting; they often feel isolated and neglected, as their parents can spare little energy or emotion for them.

Helping the bereaved family involves:

- Support and assessment through the tasks of normal mourning—most families do not need specialist counselling but benefit from general support and reassurance, supplied if possible by those who have known the family through illness
- Information—such as support groups and the Child Death Helpline. Many parents value the opportunity of talking with others who have also experienced the death of a child
- Referral for specialist bereavement counselling if needed
- Gradual withdrawal of contact.

Further reading

- ACT, Royal College of Paediatrics and Child Health. *A guide to the development of children's palliative care services*. 2nd ed. Bristol: ACT, 2003 (Tel 0117 922 1556, Fax 0117 930 4707).
- ACT, Royal College of Paediatrics and Child Health. *Palliative care for young people aged 13–14*. Bristol: ACT, 2003.
- Carson D, ed. *Medicines for children*. London: Royal College of Paediatrics and Child Health, 2003.
- Hunt A, Goldman A, Devine T, Phillips M, Fen-GBR-14 Study Group. Transdermal fentanyl for pain relief in a paediatric palliative care population. *Palliat Med* 2001;15:405–12.
- Hunt A, Goldman A, Seers K, Masstroyannopolou K, Crighton N, Moffat V. Clinical validation of the paediatric pain profile, a behavioural rating scale to assess pain in children with severe neurological and learning impairment. *Dev Child Neurol* 2004;46:9–18.
- Scott RC, Besag FM, Neville BG. Buccal midazolam and rectal diazepam for treatment of prolonged seizures in childhood and adolescence: a randomised trial. *Lancet* 1999;353:623–6.
- Wong DC, Hockenberry-Eaton M, Wilson D, Winkelstein ML, Schwartz P. *Wong's essentials of pediatric nursing*. 6th ed. St Louis, MO: Mosby, 2001:1301.

Communicating with children about death

Factors to consider

- Child's level of understanding; of illness; of death; of own situation
- Child's experience
- Family's communication pattern

Methods of communication

- Verbal
- Play
- Drama
- Art
- School work
- Stories

The loss of a child

- Multiple losses for parents:
  The child who has died
  Their dreams and hopes
  Their own immortality
  Their role as parents
- Stress on marriage
- Change in family structure
- Grief of siblings and grandparents

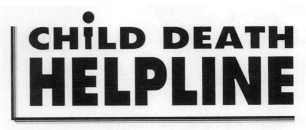

13 Communication

David Jeffrey

Why is good communication necessary?

Effective communication is essential in all clinical care. In palliative care, professionals need good communication skills to be aware of the patient's unspoken concerns. They also need to exchange information between members of the multidisciplinary team. Patients and their carers consistently identify a need for good communication with professionals, poor communication being the most common reason for complaints about doctors.

Why is communication difficult?

If communication between healthcare professionals and patients is to be improved, the reasons why communication in palliative care may be difficult must be understood.

Death remains a taboo subject and nowadays is unfamiliar to the public as most people die in hospital. Patients may have many concerns; it may not be simply the prospect of premature death but the likelihood of an undignified painful process of dying that is frightening. Doctors may feel a sense of failure as there is a tendency to blame the bearer of the bad news. Furthermore, some professionals feel unprepared to deal with the patient's emotional reactions or to admit to uncertainty.

Challenges in communication

The time of diagnosis, treatment, and recurrence of disease may be associated with considerable social and psychological morbidity, much of which remains unrecognised by healthcare professionals. It is not surprising that collusion and conspiracies of silence can develop when everyone is trying to protect the patient.

Barriers to good communication

An understanding of the factors that prevent good communication may lead to initiatives to improve it.

Lack of time
Lack of time is commonly used as a justification for inadequate communication as most clinicians have to work with unrealistic caseloads. Patients value extra time spent with them and can become more involved in decision making. Spending more time may be more efficient because it takes longer to resolve misunderstandings than to avoid them in the first instance.

Lack of privacy
Maintaining confidentiality is one way of respecting a person's autonomy and forms an essential part of a trusting relationship. In practice absolute confidentiality is hard to achieve and breaches occur in hospital and community settings.

The presence or absence of relatives can create problems of confidentiality; professionals should not assume that the patient wants the relatives to be informed. If information is judged to be highly sensitive, the patient's permission should be sought to share information with members of the multidisciplinary team on a "need to know basis."

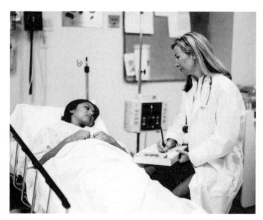

Good communication between doctor and patient is vital (photos.com)

Good communication is necessary to:
- Provide patients with information about their diagnosis, prognosis, and treatment choices to plan realistically for the future
- Make patients aware of the services that might be available for them and their carers
- Clarify the patient's priorities
- Enable a trusting relationship between the healthcare professional, patient, and family
- Reduce uncertainty and prevent unrealistic expectations while maintaining realistic hope
- Achieve informed consent
- Resolve ethical dilemmas
- Promote effective multidisciplinary teamwork

Concerns of patients
- Will the cancer come back? Fear of recurrence
- How long have I got? Fear for the future
- Why me? The search for meaning
- Am I still lovable? Body image and sexual concerns
- What can I do? Fear of loss of control
- Why won't they talk to me? Need for honesty
- Will I be a burden to others? Fear of becoming dependent
- Where is the doctor? Need for medical support

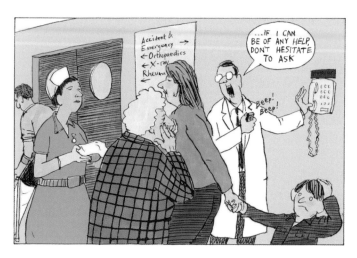

Uncertainty

Communication is particularly difficult for patients, relatives, and professionals at a time of uncertainty. Patients need to have a sense of control over their life plans. Restoring a sense of control may enable patients to feel "safe" even in a life threatening situation. Doctors should feel able to acknowledge uncertainty, be prepared to discuss patients' fears of death and dying, and assist them in setting goals for a limited future.

Embarrassment

A general reluctance in society to discuss death and dying combined with a desire not to cause patients further distress makes communication difficult. Listening is a key skill. The professional needs to convey to the patient that he or she is approachable and empathises with their suffering. Patients do not expect professionals to have answers to existential questions but they do need to have contact with another human being who is prepared to be with them and to listen to their fears.

Collusion

Collusion may arise when relatives feel that the patient would not be able to cope with bad news. This form of paternalism, which may spring from good motives, ultimately threatens patients' autonomy. It is a serious breach of confidentiality to discuss details of a case with relatives before the patient has had an opportunity to absorb the information. If collusion exists then time is needed for the healthcare professional to explore the relative's motives and feelings in a supportive way. Relatives also need to know that often the patient is fully aware of the gravity of the situation and is trying to protect them.

Maintaining hope

When patients become upset on hearing that their disease is no longer curable, their distress should be acknowledged. Given time, the patient can be encouraged to set goals other than cure—for example, relief of pain. Here healthcare professionals need to be alert for signs of clinical depression.

Anger

The doctor needs to listen to the patient's story, eliciting all their concerns. Anger should be acknowledged and not dismissed as a part of a coping process. It is therapeutic for the patient to be allowed to vent their anger without interruption. Professionals should feel free to empathise and to express feelings of regret without necessarily accepting blame.

Denial

Initially, it is common for a patient to deny the bad news and this should be expected because it is an effective coping strategy. In dealing with persisting denial, it is important to give patients an opportunity to talk as they may wish further information at a later stage. Although most patients do want to be fully informed, it is important to respect the view of the small minority who don't want further information about their diagnosis or prognosis. Patients in denial are frightened; they need patience and sensitive communication.

Not in front of the children

Children often demand information in a direct way. Older children have the same information needs as adults but require it in a form that is easily understood. Young children may need to assimilate information through the use of play, painting, videos, and books. Children need to tell their story and healthcare professionals have to be imaginative and uninhibited in helping them to articulate their distress. The natural feelings of protection should not generate situations of collusion.

Communication challenges in palliative care

- Breaking bad news
- Coping with emotional responses
- Stopping or withholding active treatments
- Avoiding collusion and promoting openness among patients, relatives, and professionals
- Discussing "Do not attempt resuscitation" orders
- Responding appropriately to a request for euthanasia
- Discussing death and dying
- Talking to children
- Communicating with colleagues

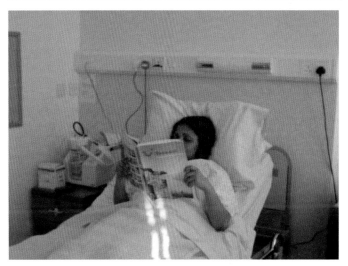

Patients may give mixed messages—reading a holiday brochure does not necessarily mean that the patient is unaware of the prognosis

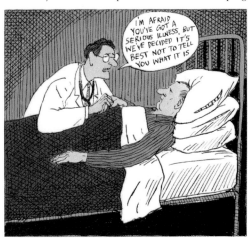

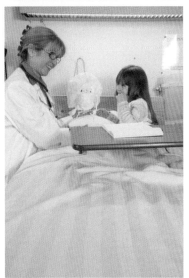

Information given to children needs to be presented in an appropriate way (photos.com)

Distancing tactics

Faced with all these challenges, it is not surprising that healthcare professionals commonly adopt distancing tactics in an effort to avoid some of the stress of communicating with patients and their families. There is a fine balance between becoming too emotionally involved with the patient's situation and adopting overt distancing tactics such as avoiding eye contact or standing at the end of the bed.

Inappropriate reassurance or cheerfulness can also inhibit a patient from raising concerns. Generally patients will want to test whether this is a doctor or nurse they can trust to discuss their fears. If their psychological cues are ignored patients quickly give up trying once they sense that the professional is not comfortable to discuss their concerns in this area.

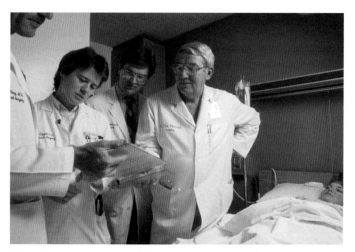

Distancing tactics, such as avoiding eye contact or standing at the end of a patient's bed, can prevent a patient discussing concerns. Reproduced with permission from Will and Deni McIntyre/Science Photo Library

Interprofessional communication

In professional training there is an emphasis on improving communication between professionals and patients, but communication between the healthcare professionals is often poor; this wastes time, threatens care of the patients, and is a source of staff stress.

Problems in interprofessional communication

Referral—Specialist palliative care services are often involved too late because of a desire to protect patients from the anticipated "distress" of referral to specialist palliative care.

Discharge planning—The provision of carefully planned care in the community requires effective communication across the hospital community interface.

Terminal care and bereavement support—Interprofessional communication may break down after the death of the patient. In one study, when deaths occurred in hospital the general practitioner was informed within 24 hours in only 16% of cases.

Organisational problems—Communication problems are a common cause of preventable disability or death in hospital patients. Research of communication systems is driven largely by technology rather than by an understanding of clinical needs.

Multidisciplinary team working—The diversity that gives a multidisciplinary team its potential for effectiveness can also make that team vulnerable if there is insufficient communication. For example, general practitioners may lose touch with patients who are being followed up in hospital clinics and feel marginalised in their care.

Communication and stress—Unsatisfactory communication lies at the heart of many of the stresses experienced by professionals working in palliative care. Such care is often uncertain; decisions have to be made with inadequate information or when advice from colleagues is conflicting. Many of the stresses reported by professionals who are caring for the dying arise from difficulties with colleagues and institutional hierarchies.

Improving communication

Breaking bad news

Breaking bad news is a process, not a single event. Kaye's steps provide a good model that can be applied to many situations of uncertainty or difficult communication.

Appropriate referral to specialist palliative care

The general practitioner is in an ideal position both to initiate the multidisciplinary team approach and to share knowledge and insights with other members of the team.

> The use of medical terms can distance professionals yet allow them to feel that they have been truthful. For example, words such as "response," "progression," and "positive" may have differing connotations in the medical and public domains

Specific problems in interprofessional communication
- Referral
- Discharge planning
- Terminal care and bereavement support
- Organisational problems
- Multidisciplinary team working
- Communication and stress

Kaye's ten steps to breaking bad news
- Preparation
- What does the patient know?
- Is more information wanted?
- Give a warning
- Allow denial
- Explain
- Listen to concerns
- Encourage feelings
- Summary and plan
- Offer availability

Assessment

General practitioners need to encourage multiprofessional primary care team working as well as enlisting the skills and knowledge of the specialist palliative care team. Role blurring is an inevitable feature of interprofessional teamwork, which can result in either competitive or collaborative relationships.

Continuity of care

It is in the patient's best interest for one doctor, usually a general practitioner, to be fully informed and responsible for continuity of the patient's medical care. The nursing care can similarly be best coordinated by the district nurse, although on occasions it may be appropriate for another member of the team to be designated the key worker.

Record keeping

Documentation is an important part of communication; the notes from the district nurses, records held by patients, and integrated care pathways are documents that can remain with the patient and facilitate interprofessional communication.

Discharge planning

General practitioners and district nurses are the key professionals responsible for medical and nursing care at home; they should be the first professionals consulted when planning a discharge from hospital.

Terminal care and bereavement support

There needs to be an efficient means of notifying the general practitioner and the primary care team of the patient's death. The team needs to identify an appropriate key worker who will be responsible for offering the family bereavement support.

Communication, conflict, and stress

Mutual respect and trust between team members leads to their corporate and individual skills being used in an optimal way. It is never helpful to be critical of colleagues in front of patients or relatives; such behaviour serves only to reduce the patient's confidence in the team. Clinical supervision, mentoring, and peer appraisal can be methods of supporting and encouraging colleagues.

Communication facilities

Team members need instruction in appropriate use of communication facilities. Voicemail, email, and mobile communication can improve support, but healthcare professionals need to think about the consequences of interrupting their colleagues and to reflect on the use of alternative approaches.

Education

A major objective of interprofessional education is fostering of mutual respect and an understanding of each other's roles.

> Honest communication is central to effective palliative care and involves more than giving information about the illness. It is concerned also with support of the patient, family, and colleagues. Information must be accurate but the manner of communication is fundamental to good practice

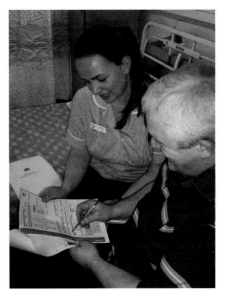

Communication between patient and professional is tailored to the individual situation

Further reading

- Buckman R. Communication in palliative care: a practical guide. In: Doyle D, Hanks GWC, Macdonald N, eds. *Oxford textbook of palliative medicine*. Oxford: Oxford University Press, 1993:47–61.
- Jeffrey D. *Cancer from cure to care*. Manchester: Hochland & Hochland, 2000.

The cartoons in this chapter are courtesy of Malcolm Willett.

14 The carers

Julia Addington-Hall, Amanda Ramirez

Most people need some care in their last months of life. Cancer patients usually experience a relatively short period of accelerating physical deterioration, while people with chronic progressive conditions such as heart failure deteriorate over a longer time frame, with unpredictable episodes of further decline. Hospitals are important providers of end of life care: more than half of all deaths take place in hospital, and 90% of all people who die have had hospital care in the last year of life. One in five deaths from causes other than cancer occurs in care homes, and many people live in these homes but die in hospital. Healthcare professionals working in institutions therefore play an important part in the care of people at the end of life.

But up to a quarter of deaths take place at home, and most people spend most of their last year of life there. Healthcare professionals have an important role here too, but support from family and friends makes all the difference to the quality of home care and to the likelihood of hospital care being avoided. These supporters are usually referred to as "informal carers," although they themselves often do not see themselves as "carers," instead seeing the care they provide as a normal part of familial relationships.

Support from family and friends

Three quarters of patients receive care at home from informal carers in the last months of life. Patients without cancer are less likely than those with cancer to have someone to care for them, reflecting their older average age at death. For people with cancer, care may be needed for weeks or months; for conditions other than cancer it may be needed for years.

Informal carers often have high levels of anxiety and depression. Lack of sleep and fatigue are common problems, and the carer's own health may suffer. Psychological morbidity while caring may be related to subsequent poor bereavement outcomes.

The degree of psychological distress is related to the amount of care patients need; the impact on carers' lives; how well the family functions under stress; the availability of social support for the carer; the carer's health status and their coping styles. Providing support for depressed, demented, or delirious patients is particularly difficult.

Carers are individuals and will respond in different ways to caregiving; there is no substitute for asking them directly about their experiences, fears, and needs. Not all the consequences of caregiving are negative: many carers report getting pleasure from being able to help someone they love. They—and the patient—will resent suggestions that the experience is wholly negative or, indeed, negative at all.

Fewer people die at home than would like to do so. Carers' views on home deaths are largely unknown. One reason for admissions is that informal caregivers are unable to continue because of deteriorations in their own health, fatigue and psychological distress, patient's increasing level of dependency, lack of confidence in their caring abilities, and the failure of health and social services to deliver appropriate care.

It is important to provide good support to informal caregivers to protect them from adverse health consequences both before and after bereavement, and to enable patients to stay at home for as long as they want. Health professionals should address carers' needs for information, practical support and advice, and psychosocial support.

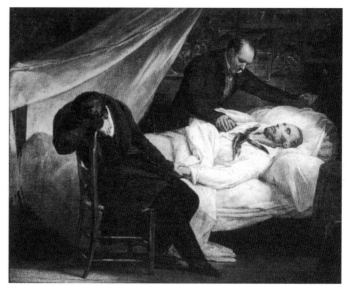

"The death of Theodore Gericault (1791–1824), with his friends Colonel Bro de Comeres and the painter" by Ary Scheffer (1795–1858). Until the start of the 20th century, most people died at home while being cared for by family and friends

---

Informal carers

- More patients want to die at home than currently do so
- Informal carers are vital to the support of patients at home
- Many informal carers are elderly and have their own health needs
- A third of caregivers provide all the informal care themselves
- Carers provide care without specialist knowledge and training, 24 hours a day, seven days a week
- Fatigue, anxiety, and depression are common among informal carers

---

Needs of informal carers

Information and education about
- The patient's diagnosis
- Causes, importance, and management of symptoms
- How to care for the patient
- Likely prognosis and how the patient may die
- Sudden changes in patient's condition, particularly those which may signal that death is approaching
- What services are available and how to access them (including in emergencies)

Support during the patient's illness
- Practical and domestic
- Respite
- Night sitters
- Psychosocial
- Financial
- Spiritual

Bereavement care
(see later article on bereavement)

Information

Information about the illness, its likely course, and what to expect as the patient deteriorates enables patients and carers to make informed decisions and reduces anxiety. It is not good practice to inform only the relatives about the patient's disease, its management, and prognosis. Exceptional circumstances may arise when patients (not relatives) clearly indicate they do not wish to discuss their illness or when patients are unable to understand the necessary information. Informing only relatives can lead to mistrust and impaired communication between patients and their relatives at a time when mutual support is most needed. Patients may choose to consult with their doctor alone, but joint consultations with both the patient and relatives avoid the problems that can arise when one or other party is informed first. Many carers report not having received all the information they wanted about the patient's illness.

Practical support and advice

Most informal carers benefit from practical instructions on how to care for patients—for example, how to lift them safely. District and palliative care nurses have an important role here, as well as in providing information on and arranging financial benefits, practical support in the home, and respite and overnight care. Availability of these resources varies widely across the UK and other countries, which places an additional burden on carers.

Psychosocial support

Mild psychological distress usually responds to emotional support from frontline health workers with effective communication skills. This involves listening to carers' concerns and fears, explaining physical and psychological symptoms, challenging false beliefs about death and dying, and helping carers reframe their experiences more positively. More severe psychological distress may benefit from specialist psychological assessment and treatment.

Healthcare professionals

Many different health professionals care for patients in their last year of life—in the community, in hospitals, and in hospices and other institutions. Some health professionals devote the whole of their working time to palliative care, while for many others it forms only a small part of their formal workload.

Psychiatric morbidity and burnout

Working in palliative care is widely believed to barrage staff with suffering and tragedy. The stress associated with caring for dying people, however, may be counterbalanced by the satisfaction of dealing well with patients and relatives. Psychiatric morbidity among palliative physicians and palliative care nurses is lower than among many other healthcare professionals.

Job stress and satisfaction

Palliative physicians and nurses report similar sources of stress as other healthcare professionals, with overload and its effect on home life being predominant. Poor management, resource limitations, and issues around care of the patients are also major sources of job stress. Palliative care nurses find difficulties in their relationships with other healthcare professionals a particular source of stress, often because their roles are poorly understood and sometimes poorly defined. Good relationships can, however, be a source of job satisfaction. Death and dying do not seem to be a major source of job stress.

Palliative physicians have significantly higher levels of job satisfaction compared with consultants working in other

---

Failing to meet informal carers' needs

- Carers are often reluctant to disclose their needs to health professionals
  Reasons for this include:
  Not wanting to focus on their own needs while the patient is still alive
  Not wanting to be judged inadequate as a carer
  Believing concerns and distress are inevitable and cannot be improved
  Not being asked relevant questions by health professional
- Attention to carers' needs will often benefit patients
- Some—perhaps many—dying patients admitted to hospital could remain at home if carers were given better support

---

Sources of support to enable informal carers to look after dying patients at home in the UK

Symptom control—General practitioners, palliative medicine domiciliary visits, district nurses, clinical nurse specialists such as Macmillan nurses
Nursing—Community nurses
Night sitting services—Marie Curie nurses, hospice at home services, district nursing services
Respite care—Hospices, community hospitals
Domestic support—Social services
Information—General practitioners, district nurses, clinical nurse specialists, voluntary organisations such as BACUP
Psychosocial support—General practitioners, district nurses, Macmillan nurses, counsellors, specific interventions for carers of dying patients
Aids and appliances—Occupational therapists
Financial assistance—Social workers, benefit officers

Risk factors for psychiatric morbidity among palliative care professionals

- For senior professionals, young age or fewer years in post
- High job stress
- Low job satisfaction
- Inadequate training in communication and management skills
- Stress from other aspects of life
- Previous psychological difficulties or family history of psychiatric problems

---

Strategies for improving mental health of professionals providing palliative care

- Maintenance of a culture of palliative care despite the shift within health care from service to business, including:
  Autonomy
  Good management
  Adequate resources, particularly with regard to workforce, so that high levels of care of patients can be maintained
- Provision of more effective training in:
  Communication
  Management skills
- Provision of effective clinical supervision that addresses the physical, psychological, social, spiritual, and communication dimensions of care of patients
- Provision of a confidential mental health service that is independent of management and covers both personal and work related problems

specialties, and palliative care nurses have significantly higher levels than most other nurses. Good relationships with patients, relatives, and staff, controlling pain and other symptoms, and improving patients' quality of life are common sources of satisfaction.

Improving the mental health of professional carers
Maintaining and improving professional carers' mental health is essential for their own wellbeing and for the quality of care that they provide for patients.

Identifying mental health problems
Some workers—particularly those with less severe mental health problems—seek advice and care from their general practitioner, a mental health colleague, or a national service. Others do not refer themselves. Often they are identified by colleagues and should be referred to a mental health specialist and to the service manager if there are concerns that care of patients may be jeopardised.

Assessment
Assessment services may be provided either within the healthcare professional's institution or, to maintain confidentiality, elsewhere by arrangement with other institutions. Such external arrangements may be particularly important for independent hospices. Assessments should be conducted by skilled mental health professionals and should include an assessment of risk to patients as well as the needs of the affected professional. Confidentiality and its limits should be discussed. It can be tempting to collude in self management, but this is a disservice to the professionals, who should be relieved of the burden of providing their own care.

Treatment
Treatment should ideally be provided outside the institution in which the professional works. The cornerstone of treatment is psychological therapy, either alone or in conjunction with psychotropic drugs. Professionals' preferences for types of treatment and their interest in exploring and understanding their problems need to be considered in the selection of the appropriate treatment(s). Psychological treatments delivered by trained staff are effective and include grief work, cognitive behaviour therapy, and behavioural and interpersonal therapy. Non-specific "counselling" and "support" are of limited benefit in managing complex severe psychological problems. Many with less severe problems report that counselling was helpful, but further evaluation is needed.

The painting by Ary Scheffer is reproduced with permission of Peter Willi and the Bridgeman Art Library, and the painting by James Hayllar is reproduced with permission of the Bridgeman Art Library.

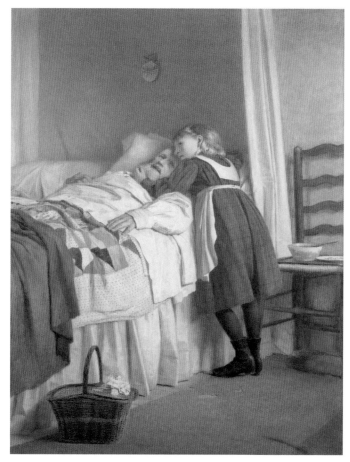

"Grandfather's little nurse" by James Hayllar (1829–1920)

Further reading
- Faulkner A, Maguire P. *Talking to cancer patients and their relatives.* Oxford: Oxford Medical Publications, 1994.
- Graham J, Ramirez AJ, Cull A, Finlay I, Hoy A, Richards MA. Job stress and satisfaction among palliative physicians. *Palliat Med* 1996;10:185–94.
- Harding R, Higginson IJ. What is the best way to help caregivers in cancer and palliative care? A systematic literature review of interventions and their effectiveness. *Palliat Med* 2003;17:63–74.
- Payne S, Ellis-Hill C, eds. *Chronic and terminal illness: new perspectives on caring and carers.* Oxford: Oxford University Press, 2001.
- Thomas C, Morris SM. Informal carers in cancer contexts. *Eur J Cancer Care* 2002;11:178–82.
- Vachon MLS. Burnout and symptoms of stress in staff working in palliative care. In: Cochinov HM, Breitbart W, eds. *Handbook of psychiatry in palliative medicine.* Oxford: Oxford University Press, 2000:303–19.

15 Chronic non-malignant disease

Marie Fallon, Joanna Chambers, Francis Dunn, Raymond Voltz, Gian Borasio, Rob George, Roger Woodruff

Introduction

All patients are entitled to good palliative care, and it is a necessary part of any practitioner's armamentarium. General clinicians and specialists therefore need a flexible and effective understanding of symptom control that can be applied diversely.

There are three main problem issues in chronic disease:

- The impact of the disease on an individual's daily living and, conversely, the possibility of improving quality of life by attending to social and practical issues
- The uncertainty of the progression of the disease and often its punctuation with exacerbations of potentially fatal complications
- Ways to modify pathology and manage symptoms.

These three issues translate into:

- Optimisation of the external environment
- Optimisation of the internal environment
- Optimisation of function and control of symptoms.

Key to the optimum way ahead for effective palliation in chronic non-malignant disease has to be effective communication between the relevant specialities. Some of the knowledge we have from working in cancer care can be transferred, though it is naive to think it is just a simple transfer of knowledge. In addition, specialists such as cardiologists, neurologists, renal physicians, and respiratory physicians will always have a key role in the palliation of most of their patients for obvious reasons.

Advanced cardiac disease

At all stages the management of cardiac disease has a substantial palliative component, and, unlike management of cancer, there are few opportunities for cure. This section focuses on palliative care in cardiac failure, as this is the final common pathway in most patients with advanced cardiac disease who do not die suddenly.

The challenge of effectively applying palliative care rests in the unpredictable course in advanced heart failure, the way in which the healthcare system is organised, and the doctor's understanding of their roles and responsibilities.

Prevalence

Cardiac failure affects 1–2% of the adult population, and the prevalence rises steeply with age (to more than 10% of those aged over 70). It is a disabling and lethal condition that also has a detrimental effect on quality of life. Up to 30% of affected patients require admission to hospital in any year (120 000 admissions annually in the UK). Mortality is higher than in many forms of cancer, with a 60% annual mortality within patients with grade 4 heart failure and an overall five year mortality of 80% in men.

Clinical aspects

There are several important similarities to and differences from cancer. One key difference, previously suspected and now confirmed, is the more linear and predictable course in cancer. In addition, it is now recognised that anaemia and pain can be regarded more as similarities than differences, and this may have implications for quality of life for patients with advanced heart failure.

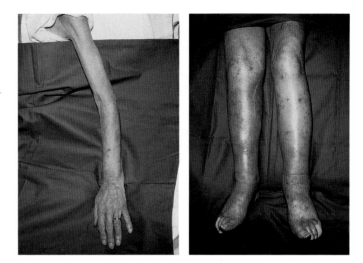

Marked muscle wasting in the arms (left) combined with oedema of the legs (right) in a patient with advanced heart failure

---

Causes of postural hypotension in advanced cardiac failure and cancer

Cardiac related
- Diuretics
- ACE inhibitors, angiotensin receptor blockers, and other vasodilators

Cancer related
- Antidepressants
- Adrenal insufficiency due to metastasis

Common to both
- Bed rest
- Coexistent disease
- Muscle wasting and poor venous tone

- Reduced fluid intake and vomiting
- Opioids

Clinical aspects of cardiac failure compared with cancer

Similarities
- Breathlessness, lethargy, cachexia
- Nausea, anorexia, abnormal taste
- Weight loss (loss of muscle mass countered by fluid retention)
- Pain
- Constipation
- Poor mobility
- Insomnia, confusion, depression
- Dizziness, postural hypotension, cough
- Jaundice, susceptibility to infection
- Polypharmacy
- Anaemia
- Abnormal liver function tests
- Fear of the future

Differences
- Predicting life expectancy is less easy
- Oedema is a more dominant feature with differing mechanism
- Patients mistakenly perceive it as a more benign condition

Management

Patients will be faced with frequent admissions to hospital. The patient's preference for management at home must be acknowledged and addressed. The heart failure liaison nurse programme pioneered in Glasgow has been shown to reduce the number of admissions by early detection and management of worsening heart failure and by ensuring that the patient's home meets all the necessary requirements for optimal home care. The patients have uniformly appreciated the support provided by this system.

Examples of requirement for hospital admission related to the home circumstances and support are:

- Need for intravenous therapy
- Persistent paroxysmal nocturnal breathlessness and orthopnoea
- Refractory oedema and fluid leakage from lower limbs
- Symptomatic postural hypotension
- Development of dysrhythmias.

Dietary advice is important and complex in that the patient may be obese or cachectic. Frequent small meals are preferable, which should be tailored to the patient's tastes. Tumour necrosis factor and interleukins are implicated in the aetiology of cachexia, and fish oils may reduce their levels. Supplements of fat soluble and water soluble vitamins may also be necessary to counteract the increased urinary loss and reduced absorption. A small amount of alcohol may help as an appetite stimulant and anxiolytic.

Reduction of fluid intake to 1500 ml a day and avoidance of excessively salty foods (but not to the extent of making food tasteless) will help to control oedema. Exercise may reduce breathlessness and improve both quality of life and psychological wellbeing. This must be tailored to each patient's needs.

Drug treatment

The main emphasis is relief from symptoms: drugs being given to improve prognosis should be reviewed.

Opioids, combined with antiemetic drugs if necessary, are useful for control of nocturnal breathlessness. Awareness of toxicity because of associated respiratory and renal insufficiency is paramount. The role of alternative opioids such as oxycodone has not been established for the easing of dyspnoea. In clinical practice, alternative opioids may be tried if side effects limit the use of morphine. Anxiolytics also have an important role, and achieving the correct balance requires individual tailoring of therapy.

Diuretics also have a key role—orally, intravenously, or in combination depending on the severity of fluid retention. However, awareness of the clinical (fatigue, nausea, and lightheadedness from postural hypotension) and biochemical features of overdiuresis is essential.

Digoxin can relieve symptoms in patients with advanced heart failure, but it is vital that symptoms of toxicity are avoided.

Angiotensin converting enzyme (ACE) inhibitors and angiotensin receptor blocking agents are beneficial, and the dose should be titrated to ensure maximum benefit without adverse effects. As many patients are volume depleted and hypotensive, small supervised test doses should be given—such as 6.25 mg of captopril or 2.5 mg of ramapril after 12–24 hours without diuretics or equivalent doses of angiotensin receptor blocking agents (definite indication for this group is cough secondary to ACE inhibitors). In patients unable to take ACE inhibitors and angiotensin receptor blocking agents, other vasodilators (such as hydralazine) might be considered, although in this situation they are of marginal value.

Home care for patients with advanced cardiac failure

- Enlist help of heart failure liaison service if available
- Assess appropriateness of the home—such as comfortable bed or recliner chair, easy access to toilet, family support
- Establish need for oxygen therapy—balance benefits and risks
- Monitor fluid status and appropriateness of diuretic treatment
- Consider normal release opioid at night (for example, oral morphine 5 mg) to ease dyspnoea but use with caution and appropriate adjustment of dose in patients with associated renal or respiratory disease
- For night sedation consider temazepam 10–20 mg, or thioridazine 10 mg or haloperidol 0.5 mg in elderly people
- Assess need for dietary advice, particularly to ensure adequate energy intake
- Ensure optimum treatment of heart failure with emphasis on symptomatic rather than prognostic benefit
- Regularly consider need for hospital admission

Management of symptoms of advanced heart failure

Breathlessness
- Oxygen
- Opioids—regular, normal release oral morphine 5 mg, or intravenous diamorphine 2.5 mg if patient is acutely distressed
- Non-drug measures such as fan, positioning, explanation, reassurance
- Diuretics, digoxin
- ACE inhibitors, angiotensin receptor blockers, and other vasodilators
- Cycle of breathlessness and panic may require an anxiolytic

Muscle wasting
- Physiotherapy
- Assess diet and energy intake

Fatigue
- Reassess drug therapy

Lightheadedness
- Check for postural hypotension
- Check for drug induced hypotension
- Exclude arrhythmia as a cause

Pain
- Analgesics—avoid NSAIDs, consider opioids as above
- Reassess anti-anginal regimen
- Non-drug measures —relaxation, TENS, hot packs, dorsal column stimulator, device therapy

Nausea, abnormal taste, anorexia
- Check drug treatments
- Check liver function
- Frequent small meals and appetite stimulants such as alcohol
- Consider metoclopramide

Oedema
- Early detection is important
- Loop diuretics—frusemide remains first choice
- Spironolactone 25 mg if tolerated. Increasing doses may help with control of oedema but watch for hyperkalaemia and painful breasts
- Restrict fluid intake to 1500–2000 ml a day
- Mild salt restriction if tolerated
- Bed rest in early stages; when patient is out of bed, raise lower limbs in a recliner chair
- Aim for weight loss of 0.5–1 kg a day
- Additional diuretic treatments may be needed, such as bendrofluazide 5 mg or metolazone 2.5 mg/day
- Monitor electrolytes

Sublingual glyceryl trinitrate may be helpful during episodes of breathlessness. Influenza and pneumococcal vaccination are worth considering despite the advanced nature of the disease.

Counselling and psychological support

Unlike for those with cancer, there is no highly developed support network for patients with end stage cardiac disease. Counselling is certainly challenging in this setting because of the high incidence of sudden death (up to 50%), as is the misconception of patients, who often underestimate the seriousness of the situation. Application of many of the principles of palliative care is needed to optimise this aspect of management.

End stage renal disease

Definitions, incidence, and prevalence

End stage renal disease or failure (ESRF) occurs when the glomerular filtration rate is insufficient to maintain health, usually when the rate is <10 ml/min. Renal replacement therapy (RRT), dialysis, or transplantation has transformed the lives of patients with ESRF, though the disease remains incurable with 10–20% of affected patients dying each year. In the past 20 years a fivefold increase in the number of patients accepted on to RRT programmes has led to a prevalence of 530 patients per million population. The median age of patients undergoing dialysis has increased from 45 to >65 in a similar time, and diabetes, once present in just 2% of patients having dialysis, is now the most common cause of ESRF in RRT programmes. This means considerable comorbidity for many patients.

Prognosis and causes of death

Age and diabetes are the key factors determining prognosis. The overall one year survival in patients with ESRF on dialysis is 84%, but the five year survival of a young person who does not have diabetes is 74% while that of someone aged >65 with diabetes is 21%. The most common cause of death is cardiovascular disease. A considerable number of patients choose to stop dialysis, and a further group opts for initial conservative management (without dialysis). Patients who choose to stop dialysis have obvious and urgent needs for terminal care; the average time to death is 10 days. A planned multidisciplinary palliative care pathway, available in some areas, will help patients who opt for conservative management, who have a less well defined time course with an average prognosis of seven months.

Management of pain and other symptoms

At least 50% of patients undergoing dialysis experience pain, which is severe for nearly half of them. Pain is often intermittent but occurs over many years and the diverse causes lead to a high incidence of neuropathic pain. Numerous factors impede good pain control. A similar approach to that used to manage cancer pain can be taken with the WHO analgesic ladder, including adjuvants where indicated. Careful monitoring for toxicity is essential because of the retention of drugs or their metabolites in patients with renal failure. The active morphine metabolite, morphine 6 glucuronide, is retained in patients with ESRF and when morphine is taken for chronic pain its retention can lead to toxicity, including cognitive impairment and myoclonus. Alternative strong opioids—such as oral hydromorphone and subcutaneous fentanyl or alfentanil and transdermal buprenorphine—are being explored. Clearance of fentanyl may be altered in patients with ESRF, though it does not have known active metabolites. Other symptoms are also

---

The future of palliation in advanced cardiac disease

- Adaptation of the role of heart failure liaison nurses to include palliative care
- Combined care from both palliative care specialists and cardiologists
- Improved understanding of mechanisms and treatment of nausea and cachexia
- Improved understanding of the role of opioids and anxiolytic agents
- Improved recognition of the need for psychological support and counselling

---

Common comorbidities in patients with ESRF

- Diabetic gastroenteropathy
- Diabetic neuropathy
- Peripheral vascular disease
- Angina
- Decubitus ulcers
- Calciphylaxis
- Falls

Causes of pain in renal failure

Concurrent comorbidity
- Peripheral vascular disease
- Diabetic neuropathy

Disease consequent on renal failure
- Amyloid related to dialysis
- Renal osteodystrophy
- Calciphylaxis

Pain related to dialysis
- Arteriovenous fistula leading to steal syndrome
- Abdominal pain from peritoneal dialysis
- Cramps and headaches

Primary renal disease
- Adult polycystic kidney disease

Barriers to good pain control

- Multiple comorbidity and multiple drug regimens
- Many causes of pain
- More than one type of pain
- Under-reporting of pain
- Altered response to drugs in renal failure
- Requirement for close monitoring
- Adverse effects of drugs
- Limb preservation despite limb ischaemia
- Pain management not a focus of training for renal physicians
- Lack of research into pharmacology of drugs in renal failure

---

Management of other symptoms related to dialysis

Optimisation of the prescription for dialysis and correction of anaemia may improve many of these symptoms

Pruritus
- Emollient cream
- Antihistamine
- Phototherapy
- Naltrexone
- $5HT_3$ antagonist

Restless legs
- Avoidance of aggravating medication
- Clonazepam
- Levodopa
- Pergolide
- Gabapentin

Cramps
- Quinine

Lethargy
- Review medication
- Manage insomnia
- Exclude depression
- Optimise nutrition
- Erythropoietin

Hypotension
- Review prescription for dialysis

Nausea
- Investigate cause and treat appropriately

common, occur over many years, and can be difficult to manage as the evidence is scarce or the remedies toxic.

Recognising the preterminal phase and end of life care

Increasing admissions to hospital and severity of pain and other symptoms with decreasing performance status often presage the terminal phase of the disease. For example, the pain of calciphylaxis, or peripheral vascular disease, with consequent amputations is known to be associated with a poor prognosis. Introducing palliative care at this stage not only enables better symptom control but can help the passage into end of life care if a decision to stop dialysis is taken. Discussion earlier in the course of disease about a person's wishes for end of life care will greatly aid decision making.

Most patients dying with ESRF die from their comorbid conditions, and their symptoms at the end of life are a continuation of those already present. Stopping dialysis does not cause pain, but pains already present are likely to continue, and joint, muscle, and skin pains may occur from reduced mobility. Shortness of breath from fluid overload may be distressing, and in the preterminal phase ultrafiltration may provide rapid relief.

Palliative care needs of patient with ESRF

Physical
- Pain
- Other symptom management
- Loss of sexual functioning
- Dietary restrictions
- Body image changes
  Haemodialysis (arteriovenous fistulae; vascular access lines)
  Peritoneal dialysis (abdominal distension; catheters)

Social
- Loss of employment
- Change in role
- Dependence on carers and machines
- Time spent on dialysis
- Loss of freedom for travel

Psychological
- Depression
- Guilt
- Anxiety
- Uncertainty

Spiritual
- Facing own and others death
- Cultural: ESRF is more common in Afro-Caribbean people
- Finding meaning out of the experience

Respiratory disease

While formal lung function tests are useful, with palliation the objective is to make the patient feel better. Therefore, the most practical and pragmatic way of measuring the effectiveness of treatment is to score breathlessness or cough on a digital or analogue scale or by measuring walking distance. An important exception is hypoxaemia. This is the final common path of respiratory failure and on the way leads to several debilitating compensatory mechanisms. The objective should be to maintain oxygen saturation above 90%, which will minimise the likelihood of developing cor pulmonale. Difficulties may arise in patients with impaired ventilatory drive who depend in part on their hypoxia rather than hypercapnia. Apart from the apocryphal "blue bloater" with COPD, impaired drive is a common feature of the neuromuscular diseases.

Good care

Good general care is central to maintaining quality of life, social productivity, and a sense of self. Nutrition is often an early casualty of breathlessness as eating requires a lot of effort. In turn, this compounds muscle weakness together with falling

---

Modified WHO analgesic ladder for patients with ESRF

All steps
- Adjuvants* as indicated by type of pain
- NSAIDs†

Step 1
- Paracetamol 1 g four times a day

Step 2‡
- Tramadol up to 50 mg four times a day

Step 3§

Oral route:
- Hydromorphone 1.3 mg every four to six hours and as needed
- Morphine 5–10 mg every four to six hours and as needed
- If patient is on sufficient regular strong opioid, consider "offloading" background dose to fentanyl patch or buprenorphine patch; always titrate to patch and watch for change in pain or clinical condition
- Subcutaneous route: fentanyl, alfentanil, or hydromorphone

* Clonazepam is a useful adjuvant for neuropathic pain in ESRF, titrate against toxicity.

† NSAIDs should not be used in a patient who is not receiving dialysis.

‡ Tramadol is preferable to codeine for step 2 as there may be idiosyncratic occurrence of respiratory depression with codeine. Maximum 24 hour dose of tramadol is 200 mg. Dihydrocodeine should be avoided.

§ All strong opioids should be monitored carefully; remember that pain and the patient's clinical condition often change rapidly.

End of life care

- General considerations
  Acknowledgement and agreement of goals of care
  Discontinuation of unnecessary investigations, monitoring, and non-palliative medication
- Continue regular medication for symptom relief
- When parenteral drugs are required
  Analgesia: use subcutaneous fentanyl or alfentanil* as strong opioid of choice
  Antiemesis: can continue cyclizine †, haloperidol, metoclopramide‡, or levomepromazine§ if they are already successful
  Sedation: midazolam¶
- Anticipatory prescribing with as needed subcutaneous medication, which can be put in a 24 hour syringe driver as clinically indicated:
Pain: fentanyl 12.5–25 µg as needed or alfentanil 0.1–0.2 mg up to hourly
  Retained respiratory secretions: hyoscine butylbromide 20 mg immediately and up to every four hours
  Terminal agitation distress: midazolam 2.5–5 mg up to hourly
  Nausea and vomiting: levomepromazine 5 mg up to every eight hours

*In patients who have never taken opioids, successful pain relief can be achieved with low doses—for example, 150–200 µg fentanyl/24 hours—without excess sedation.

†Avoid if possible because patients with renal failure tend to have dry mouth.

‡Do not exceed 40 mg/24 hours.

§Increased sensitivity, very low doses usually suffice.

¶Increased sensitivity, use 50–75% of normal dose.

Optimising lung function

- Physiological assessment (tests according to pathology)
- Go by measures of breathlessness or exercise tolerance
- Measures of lung function are only guidelines as to palliative efficacy
- Manage hypoxaemia (maintain O_2 saturation above 90%):
  Long term O_2 therapy
  Exercise O_2
- Minimise infection
- Specific interventions on specialist advice—for example:
  Nocturnal ventilatory support
  Surgical volume reduction in COPD

fitness. Equally, bowel care matters: constipation means more effort in defecation and diaphragmatic splinting, both of which worsen symptoms unnecessarily.

Rehabilitation

Fear in any form reduces a patient's tolerance to distress from symptoms. Explanations about the mechanisms of breathing and how to control and "ride" an episode of breathlessness, together with the assurance that they will not suffocate, help patients to control breathlessness.

Practically speaking, exercise programmes for muscle conditioning generally, and the respiratory muscles in particular, may be beneficial. Training in certain types of breathing and developing efficient and effective patterns during exercise and recovery are important. Techniques such as breathing with pursed lips and the use of accessory muscles and posture to relieve distress in diseases with obstructive components help to reduce lung volume and the sensation of breathlessness. Interestingly, cold air on the face, by activating the primitive diving reflex, reduces ventilation and breathlessness. A hand held fan may be a useful emergency measure and can be kept in a pocket or handbag.

Effective cough (huffing) is important for patients with excessive secretions (such as in cystic fibrosis, bronchiectasis, etc) as is the use of postural drainage as a prophylaxis against the chronic bronchial damage of recurrent infections. These dimensions of care are best delivered by respiratory physiotherapists or nurse specialists in specific clinics as part of a multidisciplinary team.

Medical interventions

Respiratory diseases usually affect several parts of the respiratory system and control axis. One should always consider each element in turn to ensure that patients have the best chance of maintained function.

Airways obstruction

Bronchodilators—Anticholinergics and β agonists remain the mainstay of treatment and should be used as long as patients are able to take them. Spacer devices are just as good if not better than nebulisers as drugs can penetrate to the smaller airways. Sustained release theophyllines may benefit some.

Steroids—If patients have not had trials of steroid, they should be given prednisolone 30 mg for two weeks with review. If there is no substantial improvement in symptoms or exercise tolerance, they should be stopped. If there is benefit, then weaning to inhaled steroids is preferable to minimise the effects on muscle strength. Steroids are also likely to boost the appetite and may break an anorexic cycle if that is in process.

Anti-inflammatories and antibiotics—Nebulised or oral NSAIDs such as ibuprofen may be effective in reducing airways damage from chronic infection. In patients with bronchiectasis or cystic fibrosis, however, control may justify long term use of antibiotics or rotations either orally or via nebuliser. This should be managed by specialists. Steroids should not be used, except in patients with bronchopulmonary aspergillosis.

Managing cough

It is as important to promote effective expectoration as to reduce irritating or excessive cough. Conventionally in palliative care the priority is to reduce secretions and cough as patients are entering the phase of active dying. This is entirely right, but in chronic respiratory diseases persisting cough may be down to ineffectiveness in clearing secretions.

Non-medical support and care

General
- Explanation
- Nutrition
- Practical aids in the home

Rehabilitation (specialist help from respiratory physiotherapists or nurses necessary)
- Exercise programmes for fitness and respiratory muscle conditioning
- Effective cough (huffing) when secretions are excessive

Effective breathing patterns—for example:
- Purse lip in obstruction
- Slow expiratory phase to help abort panic attacks
- Breath control during exercise
- Cold air on the face from a hand fan reduces ventilation

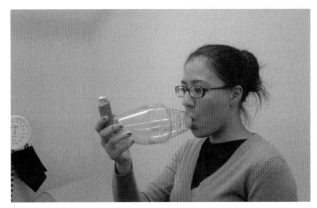

A spacer device can facilitate the use of inhalers in breathless patients in any setting. Reproduced from Rees J, Kanabar D. *ABC of asthma.* 5th ed. Blackwell Publishing: Oxford, 2006

Managing cough and secretions
- Improving effectiveness
- Reducing viscosity of secretions to aid the mucociliary escalator
- Nebulised saline
- Antibiotics if appropriate
- N-acetyl cysteine, etc (seek specialist advice)
- Effective physiotherapy
- Training in forced expiratory "huffing"
- Postural drainage
- Mini-tracheostomy for suction should be considered with specialist advice
- Treat any bronchospasm or infection
- Opioids
- Anticholinergics by inhalation, mouth, or injection

Opioids

It is almost axiomatic in general training that, because there is a known dose dependent reduction in ventilation with opioids, they are dangerous and potentially life threatening. It is not as simple as this in patients with chronic disease.

- Firstly, the reduction in respiratory drive in breathless patients is a potent source of symptom relief and may allow slower and deeper breaths that reduce dead space ventilation and make breathing more efficient.
- Secondly, studies at the end of life show that there is no shortening of expected survival time in patients in whom opioids or sedatives are being titrated up for optimum symptom relief.
- Opioids remain the most effective antitussives and should not be withheld for the above reasons either. Though it has not been proved, there is a general view that normal release opioids such as Oramorph or Sevredol are better for breathlessness, and doses should start at 2.5 mg every four hours titrated against breathlessness or cough.
- Finally, as with most chronic disease, pain is present in about two thirds of patients and should be managed as in any other condition, and opioids if indicated must not be withheld. If this is a source of anxiety, then specialist palliative care physicians or nurses should be involved.

Sedatives

Sedatives have a mixed press in the management of breathlessness and results of studies are inconclusive. Some patients, however, may benefit, and consideration should always be given to a therapeutic trial. Benzodiazepines in low dose—for example, diazepam 2 mg or lorazepam 0.5 mg every eight hours or buspirone 20 mg a day—will be suitable. When anxiety or panic attacks are a prominent feature, sedative should be used without hesitation.

Amyotrophic lateral sclerosis/motor neurone disease

Neurological disorders are among the leading causes of death in the Western world and require specific knowledge in palliative care. As an example, we will concentrate on palliative care for people with amyotrophic lateral sclerosis (ALS) or motor neurone disease.

ALS is the most common degenerative motoneurone disorder in adults. The mean age at onset is 58 years and the average duration of disease is three to four years. There is no curative treatment; the only approved drug (riluzole) prolongs life by about three months. The main symptoms are directly or indirectly due to the condition. Palliative care starts with the communication of the diagnosis and goes all the way to bereavement counselling, involving a large number of different professionals. In the UK, around three quarters of inpatient palliative care/hospice units are involved in the care of patients with ALS.

Control of symptoms

Muscle weakness should be managed by regular exercise, never to the point of fatigue, and by the use of appropriate aids to maintain independence and mobility (such as ankle-foot orthosis, wheelchair, aids for dressing and eating, etc).

Dysphagia should first be treated by an adjustment in diet (recipe books are available from several associations). Specific swallowing techniques can help to prevent aspiration. A PEG is usually well tolerated, provided the forced vital capacity is >50% at the time of introduction. At later stages, PEG insertion should be performed under non-invasive ventilation.

> The only way to be sure that either opioids or sedatives are unsuitable is to conduct a closely monitored therapeutic trial, and if there is serious concern that respiratory drive may be compromised, then it is justified to admit the patient to monitor the introduction

Symptoms due to ALS (either as a direct consequence of motoneuronal degeneration or indirectly as a consequence of the primary symptoms)

Directly:
- Weakness and atrophy
- Fasciculations and muscle cramps
- Spasticity
- Dysarthria
- Dysphagia
- Dyspnoea
- Pathological laughing/crying

Indirectly:
- Psychological disturbances
- Sleep disturbances
- Constipation
- Drooling
- Thick mucous secretions
- Symptoms of chronic hypoventilation
- Pain

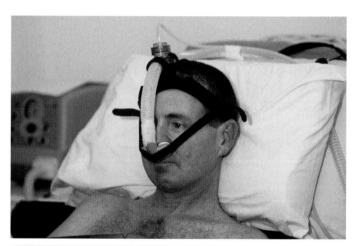

Man with motor neurone disease on a ventilator (reproduced with permission of Dr P Marazzi/Science Photo Library)

Dysarthria can lead to a complete loss of oral communication. Speech therapy is helpful at the beginning. Modern computer technology offers several options for communication even in advanced stages.

Dyspnoea is the most severe symptom in ALS. At the onset of dyspnoea, chest physiotherapy is helpful. Dyspnoeic attacks with pronounced anxiety can be treated with sublingual lorazepam (0.5–1 mg). Chronic dyspnoea may require morphine (2.5–5 mg orally or 1–2 mg subcutaneously or intravenously every four hours). Titration of the dose of morphine against the clinical effect will rarely lead to a life threatening respiratory depression. Months to years before terminal respiratory failure, symptoms of chronic nocturnal hypoventilation ensue, which may considerably hamper the patient's quality of life. Non-invasive intermittent ventilation via a mask is efficient and cost effective in alleviating these symptoms.

Thick mucous secretions result from a combination of diminished fluid intake and reduced coughing pressure. N-acetylcysteine may help. Suction is usually not fully effective unless performed via a tracheostomy. Physical therapy with vibration massage may help initially. Both manually assisted coughing techniques and mechanical insufflation-exsufflation can assist in extracting excess mucus from the airway.

Pathological laughing or crying occurs in up to 50% of patients and can be disturbing in social situations. Physicians should ask about it and point out that it responds well to medication.

Pain is common in advanced stages, is often musculoskeletal in origin, and should be treated according to the WHO analgesic ladder. Other symptoms can also be relieved by appropriate medication. For antispasticity drugs, the patient has to titrate the dose against the clinical effect as a moderate degree of spasticity is usually better for mobility than a fully flaccid paresis.

Information on the terminal phase

At the onset of dyspnoea or symptoms of chronic hypoventilation or when the forced vital capacity drops below 50%, patients should be offered information about the terminal phase as at this point they fear that they will "choke to death." Describing the mechanism of terminal hypercapnic coma and the resulting peaceful death during sleep can relieve this fear.

Terminal phase

More than 90% of patients die peacefully, mostly in their sleep. The death process usually begins with the patients slipping from sleep into coma due to increasing hypercapnia. If signs of dyspnoea develop, morphine should be administered beginning with 2.5–5 mg (oral, subcutaneous, or intravenous) every four hours. If restlessness or anxiety is present, sublingual lorazepam (start with 1–2.5 mg) or oral or subcutaneous midazolam (start with 1–2 mg) should be given. Most patients with ALS want to die at home. This can best be achieved through early enrolment in a hospice or palliative care programme.

A list of associations for patients with ALS can be found at www.alsmndalliance.org; a list of ALS centres is at www.wfnals.org

HIV/AIDS

The natural course of infection with HIV is that it evolves over a period of years into AIDS, which is uniformly fatal. The estimates published by UNAIDS show the enormity of the pandemic, reflecting mortality and morbidity of catastrophic proportions.

Symptoms of chronic nocturnal hypoventilation

- Daytime fatigue and sleepiness, concentration problems
- Difficulty falling asleep, disturbed sleep, nightmares
- Morning headache
- Nervousness, tremor, increased sweating, tachycardia
- Depression, anxiety
- Tachypnoea, dyspnoea, phonation difficulties
- Visible efforts of auxiliary respiratory muscles
- Reduced appetite, weight loss, recurrent gastritis
- Recurrent or chronic upper respiratory tract infections
- Cyanosis, oedema
- Vision disturbances, dizziness, syncope
- Diffuse pain in head, neck, and extremities

Drugs to treat symptoms in ALS (in order of recommendation)

Drug	Dose*
Fasciculations and muscle cramps	
Mild:	
Magnesium	5 mmol 3–4 times/day
Vitamin E	400 IE twice/day
Severe:	
Quinine sulphate	200 mg twice/day
Carbamazepine	200 mg twice/day
Phenytoin	100 mg 3–4 times/day
Spasticity	
Baclofen	10–80 mg per 24 hours
Tizanidine	6–24 mg per 24 hours
Tetrazepam	100–200 mg per 24 hours
Drooling	
Glycopyrrolate	0.1–0.2 mg subcutaneous/intramuscular times/day
Transdermal hyoscine patches	1–2 patches/72 hours
Amitriptyline	10–150 mg/72 hours
Botulinum toxin injections (for refractory cases)	
Pathological laughing/crying	
Amitriptyline	10–150 mg/24 hours
Fluvoxamine	100–200 mg/24 hours

*Usual range of adult daily dose; some patients may require higher doses of, for example, antispastic medication.

UNAIDS estimates of the HIV/AIDS epidemic (December 2005)

People newly infected in 2005	4.9 million
Total number of people with HIV/AIDS	40.3 million
AIDS deaths in 2005	3.1 million
Total deaths from AIDS since 1981	25 million
www.unaids.org	

ABC of palliative care

In developed countries, the introduction of combination therapies with reverse transcriptase and protease inhibitors (referred to as highly active antiretroviral therapy or HAART) during the mid-1990s had profound effects on the clinical features and outlook for patients with HIV/AIDS. HAART led to a lengthening of the time to the development of AIDS and significantly improved survival after the diagnosis of AIDS.

The clinical course of AIDS is characterised by the occurrence of opportunistic infections and constitutional symptoms related to AIDS (weight loss, fever, and diarrhoea). Some patients will develop related malignancy or related neurological disease. Patients suffer increasingly frequent infections that may become less responsive to therapy and from which they recover progressively less well. The clinical course of AIDS can be broadly grouped into four phases that show the gradual shift in the goals of treatment with progression of the disease.

Palliative care and AIDS

Palliative care for patients with AIDS is about quality of life and is directed at the alleviation of pain and physical symptoms as well as the assessment and management of psychosocial problems. It also involves care and support of family members or partners, including bereavement follow-up. It requires a holistic approach to care and is best provided by a well coordinated multidisciplinary team. It must be provided in a manner that shows respect for the individual patient—their dignity, their culture, their choices and wishes regarding treatment, and their goals and unfinished business.

The timing and delivery of palliative care to patients with AIDS is complicated by the occurrence of clinical episodes requiring acute interventions. There should be palliative care involvement long before the terminal phase of the illness, complementary to other medical care and not sequential to it. Even though HIV infection is incurable and ultimately fatal, its various manifestations are eminently treatable, and it is appropriate to provide pain relief, symptom control, and psychosocial support to patients with advanced disease while they continue to pursue treatment to control the disease.

Pain and symptom control

Management involves identifying and treating the underlying cause of symptoms, when possible and clinically appropriate. In AIDS, this may include the use of several different methods of treatment, including treatments to control disease. All palliative treatment should be appropriate to the stage of the patient's disease and the prognosis, although the fluctuating course of the condition can make decisions about appropriate therapy quite difficult.

The high incidence of cognitive impairment and dementia in the later stages makes advance care planning important, and matters of guardianship and wills should be dealt with as early as possible.

Psychosocial problems

In developed countries, most patients with AIDS are homosexual men, injecting drug users (IDUs), or from immigrant or other minority groups. In addition to dealing with a life threatening illness, they bring with them myriad psychosocial problems. Treatment includes support and counselling and the provision of appropriate services, all of which need to be done in a culturally appropriate and sensitive manner.

Clinical course of AIDS

Early stage
- Recent diagnosis of AIDS
- Good response to antiretroviral therapy and treatment of infections
- Normal activities, work

Progressive stage
- Increasing number and frequency of infections
- Progressive weight loss, increasing fatigue
- Capable of partial activity, work

Advanced stage
- Increasing or constant infections with poor response to treatment
- Fatigue and debility seriously affect daily function
- Stop active treatment; the goal of treatment is now comfort

Terminal stage
- Totally dependent
- Death can be anticipated within days to a few months
- Care is entirely comfort orientated

Prevalence of symptom in patients with AIDS

Symptom	Prevalence (%)
Anorexia/weight loss	91
Fatigue/weakness	77
Pain	63
Incontinence (urine/stool)	55
Shortness of breath	48
Confusion	43
Nausea/GI upset	35
Cough	34
Anxiety/depression	32
Loss of vision	25
Skin breakdown	24
Constipation	24
Oedema	23
Psychological issues	18
Skin problems	17
Seizures	16
Fever	13
Potential for skin breakdown	4
Agitation	1

From Casey House Hospice, Toronto.

Treatment of pain and symptoms related to AIDS

Disease specific therapy
- Treatment of opportunistic infections: antimicrobial drugs
- Anticancer therapy for related cancer: radiotherapy, chemotherapy
- HAART

Symptomatic therapy
- Analgesics, antiemetics

Psychosocial interventions
- Non-pharmacological therapies—for example, relaxation, meditation
- Management of anxiety, depression: medications, supportive psychotherapy
- Supportive counselling

Patients from the male homosexual community, IDUs, and immigrants from areas where HIV is heterosexually endemic may have experienced many previous bereavements as friends and family members died from AIDS, which will heighten their distress as their disease progresses.

Terminal care

The clinical features of terminal AIDS are not very different to those of cancer, although the duration of the terminal phase may be more variable. The last few days of life involve debility and dependency, semiconsciousness, and poor oral intake and may feature generalised pain, restlessness, and rattling respiration. These symptoms respond to standard measures, including subcutaneous analgesics, anxiolytics, and anticholinergics.

Further reading

- O'Neill JF, Selwyn PA, Schietinger H, eds. *A clinical guide to supportive and palliative care for HIV/AIDS*. Washington DC: HIV/AIDS Bureau, US Department of Health and Human Services, 2003.
- Pratt RJ. *HIV and AIDS*. 5th ed. London: Edward Arnold, 2002.
- Woodruff R, Glare P. HIV/AIDS in adults. In: Doyle D, ed. *Oxford textbook of palliative medicine*. 3rd ed. Oxford: Oxford University Press, 2003.

Examples of psychosocial problems

Psychological
- Fear, anxiety
- Depression
- Demoralisation
- Cognitive impairment, dementia
- Alcohol or substance abuse
- Multiple bereavements
- Physical disfigurement
- Suicidal ideation

Spiritual or existential
- Questions of meaning and purpose
- Questions about religion

Social
- Separation from biological family (homosexual men)
- Poor social networks (IDUs)
- Poor housing, homelessness
- Poor financial resources
- Confidentiality

Cultural
- Homosexual men
- IDUs
- Immigrants' attitudes to disease and health care

16 Community palliative care

Keri Thomas

Few things in general practice are more important and more rewarding than enabling a patient to die peacefully at home. For GPs, district nurses, and others in the primary health care team (PHCT), this is an important and intrinsic part of their work. They deliver most palliative care to patients and generally do this in a sound and effective way, especially when they are backed by appropriate specialist support. People now live longer with serious illness, with most of the time spent living "normally" at home, so providing good community based care is vital. Sensitively facing the reality of dying and making a plan for the final stage of life is as important in end of life care as planning for pregnancy and labour are in antenatal or early life care. Yet this pre-emptive planning is often omitted, resulting in a tendency towards reactive, crisis led care that does not always meet the needs of dying patients. The paradox is that although most of the final year of life is spent at home, and most people would choose to die there, increasingly most people still die in hospital. The excessive numbers of hospital admissions are due mainly to:

- Unresolved symptom control
- A breakdown in provision of home care services—for example, lack of nursing/night sitters
- Lack of support for carers.

Many more patients would prefer to die at home than are currently able to do so, and a hospital death is more likely to occur in particular groups of patients, such as the poor, the elderly, solitary women, and those with a long illness. Many choose to die in hospices (although currently only about 17% of patients with cancer and 4% of all patients die there), and many hospice outreach teams extend specialist support to the home, working closely with community teams.

Increased advanced care planning—supporting more people to cope well at home and improving the quality of palliative care provided by generalists in the community, in hospital, and in care homes—would increase the numbers of people who are able to die where they choose and prevent some unnecessary hospital admissions, thereby increasing inpatient bed capacity.

The most important challenge we face in service provision, therefore, is to enable more people to live well and die well in the place and in the manner of their choosing. Practically this means to optimise the quality and reliability of palliative care services provided by all and to reduce crises and unnecessary hospital admissions.

Home care

Ninety percent of the final year of life is spent at home, no matter where the patient eventually dies. Home is a special place, a state of mind, a place to be ourselves most fully. It represents life, activity, self determination, and retaining control, rather than illness, passivity, and the "patient mode" of inpatient care. The preferred place of care may seem to change nearer death; this may be by default—for example, when patients or their carers feel unable to cope, for relief of symptoms, the fear of being a burden, and sometimes conflict between the patient and the carer's choice. But it has to be questioned whether this is real "choice" or a response to practicalities by default—with better planning and support can a change sometimes be averted? Many people would choose to spend most time at home but to die in a

---

Key facts around palliative care in the community

- 90% of the final year of life is spent at home
- Most people prefer to die at home, but the number who choose a hospice is increasing
- The home death rate is low (23% for patients with cancer, 19% for all deaths)
- The hospital death rate is high (55% for patients with cancer, 66% of all deaths)
- 21% of those aged over 65 years in care homes (nursing and residential homes)
- Death in hospital is more likely if patients are poor, elderly, have no carers, are female, or have a long illness
- Each GP has about 30–40 patients with cancer at one time
- District nurses coordinate most palliative care in the home
- Primary palliative care is optimised by formalised specialist support
- Less support is available for patients with illnesses other than cancer and their carers and GPs
- Gaps in community care include control of symptoms, support of carers, 24 hour nursing care, night sitters, access to equipment, out of hours support
- Improving community palliative care services (including care homes) has an impact on hospitals and hospices
- The average length of stay in a hospice is now two weeks, 98% of patients have cancer and 50% of patients in hospices will be discharged
- Enabling patients to die in the place of their choice can have a positive effect on the family's bereavement

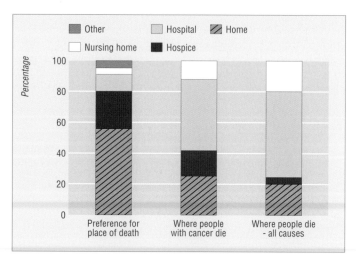

Priorities for end of life care in England, Wales, and Scotland (data from Cecily Saunders Foundation and National Council for Palliative Care)

hospice, an appropriate choice for many—yet many of our hospice services would struggle currently to meet this preference, especially for patients without cancer.

With the increase in advanced directives or living wills, it is more important than ever to have these difficult discussions with patients and their families early on and together form an advanced care plan including decisions about their preferences, such as place of care, which should be noted and communicated to others. Other areas to cover include a nominated proxy, do not resuscitate (DNR) decisions, what patients would or would not like to happen, what to do in a crisis, and special requests—for example, organ donation. This enables a greater sense of self determination and control and better planning of care based on the needs of the patient.

Time is short for the dying. Towards the end of life the pace of change may be rapid, and without good planning and proactive management, the speed of events can catch out the best of us. Enabling dying patients to remain at home involves a close collaboration of many people, services, and agencies, both generalist and specialist and, at best, an agreed system or managed plan of care (such as the gold standards framework). A bewildering number of people can become involved, sometimes causing a confusing mismatch of services and adding to the trauma of the dying process. Patients and carers appreciate the continuity, coordination, and ongoing relationship with their primary care team or specialist provider.

So within community palliative care there is a pressing need for active anticipatory management, coordination, and "orchestration" of services to enable good home care for the dying. Although GPs may feel pressurised by time constraints, the primary care team, particularly the district nurses, are in a key role to perform this function, and often they are the mainstay of care at this most crucial time. This is in line with the "cradle to grave" concepts inherent in primary care; knowledge of context and community and of continuing supportive relationship and care of the dying is close to the heart of most people working in primary care. As Gomas (1993) said "Palliative care at home embraces what is most noble in medicine: sometimes curing, always relieving, supporting right to the end."

The needs of dying patients

Palliative care services should respond to the needs of patients and carers and deliver to their agenda. This requires a holistic assessment, including non-medical psychosocial issues. In general, patients want to remain as free from symptoms as possible and to feel secure and supported, with good information and proactive planning. This allows the continued journeying to other important and deeper levels involved in the dying process—for example, loving relationships, retaining dignity, self worth, spiritual peace. Various studies confirm what is required of healthcare professionals by dying patients and their carers. Good communication and information figure largely—for example, clear advice on what to do in an emergency, what to expect— and also the steadfast continuity of relationships, the "being there," as "companions on the journey" with our patients. This trusted relationship and supportive role should never be underestimated.

Support from councillors or psychologists is sometimes available, which may smooth the transition and mental adaptation required in coming to terms with dying. Social services need to be involved for advice on financial benefits, continuing care services, respite, and social care. The DS1500

Needs and requests of patients and carers

Requirements of patients and carers at home
- Nursing and medical care
- Good symptom control
- Information—for example, what to expect/who to phone in a crisis
- Practical advice/help/equipment
- Good liaison across boundaries
- Continuity of relationship with clinicians
- Social care—for example, continuous care funding, etc
- Support for carers—night sitters, Marie Curie nurses, etc
- Carers' needs assessed
- Preparing families for a death
- Information on what to do after death

What patients especially appreciate from their GPs
- Continuity of relationship
- Being listened to
- Opportunity to ventilate feelings
- Being accessible
- Effective symptom control

Key components of best practice in community palliative care

Use of the gold standards framework, NICE Guidance on Supportive and Palliative Care, Generalist Palliative Care www.nice.org.uk

- Patients with needs for palliative care are identified according to agreed criteria and a management plan discussed within the multidisciplinary team
- These patients and their carers are regularly assessed with agreed assessment tools
- Anticipated needs are noted, planned for, and addressed
- Needs of patients and carers are communicated within the team and to specialist colleagues, as appropriate
- Preferred place of care and place of death are discussed and noted, and measures taken to comply when possible
- A named person in the practice team orchestrates coordination of care
- Relevant information is passed to those providing care out of hours, and drugs that may be needed left in the home
- A protocol for care in the dying phase is followed, such as the Liverpool care pathway for the dying patient
- Carers are educated, enabled, and supported, which includes the provision of specific information, financial advice, and bereavement care
- Audit, reflective practice, development of practice protocols, and targeted learning are encouraged as part of personal, practice, and primary care organisation/NHS trust development plans

The term "psychosocial" care includes the psychological, social, spiritual, and practical needs of the patient and carers, all of which need to be assessed and addressed where possible

attendance allowance form should be used by primary care teams to enable speedy additional funding for those in the last six months of life. Spiritual needs may be hard to assess and personally challenging but vital to enable people to move towards a peaceful conclusion of their lives. Referral to the appropriate spiritual advisor and awareness of ethnic differences in this diverse multicultural nation is all part of good care. Practical needs include equipment such as mattresses, wheelchairs, commodes, syringe driver, and home modifications such as external key boxes and handrails, etc.

Primary care team response

Working as a team, the PHCT can provide continuous and coordinated supportive care in the community. Early referral to the district nursing service is preferred, allowing time for a full assessment of the needs of the patient and carer, early referral to other services, ordering of equipment, and time to develop a relationship with the patient and carer as advocate and "key worker"' before later deterioration.

Out of hours care

Particular attention should be paid to improving the continuity of care out of hours, which accounts for about 75% of the week. Without this vital aspect, all the good work of primary care can be instantly dismantled, and the patient can be admitted to hospital in crisis, possibly to remain there until death. In the UK, changes in the contracted out of hours cover might threaten the continuity of care for dying patients. With better proactive management and the use of an agreed protocol, a handover form, and good access to drugs, however, these situations could be avoided.

Support for family and carers

Support for the family and carer can be one of the most important aspects of the holistic care provided by primary care teams, backed up by hospice support if available. Carer breakdown is often the key factor in prompting institutionalised care for dying patients. Carers should be included as full members of the team, enabled, forewarned, informed, and taught to care for the dying patient to the level desired. This has consequences for the carer in bereavement, with a greater satisfaction that the patient's final wishes were fulfilled and fewer "if only . . ." regrets later. The toll of caring for a dying person can be considerable in both physical and emotional terms; many carers are elderly and infirm themselves and there is an increased morbidity and mortality of carers in bereavement.

In some surveys of both patients and families, the carer's anxiety is rated alongside the patient's symptoms as the most severe problem. There is resounding evidence that without support from family and friends it would be impossible for many patients to remain at home.

This is one issue where evidence confirms that primary care can make a real and valued difference. Many carers, however, feel that GPs do not understand their needs, and in turn many GPs and district nurses feel they lack the relevant time, resources, and training to take a more proactive role. The primary care team, however, is in a key position to help, both personally and in coordinating services. Separate assessment and practical support for carers is therefore required and, with support from social services and self help groups, carers are then more likely to be able to withstand the pressure. Those without carers may struggle even more, and they present particular difficulties for primary care in an age of increasing solitary living.

Carers need time to ask questions, to discuss decisions, to help relieve their anxiety, and to create a better understanding

A protocol for out of hours (OOH) palliative care

- Communication:
  Handover form to OOH provider
  Inform others—for example, hospice
  Does the carer know what to do in a crisis?
- Carer support:
  Coordinate pre-emptive care—for example, night sitters
  Give written information to carers
  Emergency support—for example, rapid response team
- Medical support:
  Anticipated management in handover form
  Crisis pack, guidelines, etc, and ongoing teaching
  24 hour specialist advice available—for example, from hospice
- Drugs/equipment:
  Leave anticipated drugs in home
  Palliative care bags available
  On-call stocked pharmacists

Improve access to palliative care drugs

Suggested list of drugs to be left in the home of every palliative care patient
- Diamorphine
- Cyclizine/haloperidol
- Midazolam
- Hyoscine butylbromide/hydrobromide/glycopyrronium

Adapted from Thomas K, *Eur J Pall Care* 2000;7:22–5.

> Carer breakdown is a crucial and sometimes unrecognised issue, and carers have their own separate needs for assessment and support. This important factor must be addressed if any impact is to be made on home based palliative care (see chapter 14)

Supporting carers—what primary care can do

- Acknowledge carers, what they do, and the problems they have
- Assess health and welfare of the carer as well as the patient
- Treat carers as you would other team members and listen to their opinions
- Include them in discussions about the patient
- Flag informal carer's notes, so other health workers are aware of their circumstances
- Give carers a choice about which tasks they undertake
- Provide information about the condition
- Provide information about being a carer and support and benefits available
- Provide information about local services available for patient and carer
- Ensure that services and equipment provided
- Liaise with other services—be an advocate for the carer
- Ensure staff are informed about the needs and problems of informal carers
- Respond quickly and sympathetically to crisis situations
- Give or arrange training—for example, in lifting and moving, giving medication, etc
- Confide in and listen to patients/carers—let them express their needs and support them
- Suggest coping strategies, both internal (faith, positive attitude, etc) and external (social networks)
- Development of a bereavement protocol and raising awareness of bereaved patients in practice teams
- Assemble a list of local contacts for bereavement support

of what is happening. It is often helpful to rehearse with the carer what to do in certain situations, such as if the patient has uncontrolled symptoms or when the patient dies.

Together with the provision of back up 24 hour contact details, this will enhance a sense of security and confidence and reduce the chance of crisis calls. Management plans, advanced directives, and do not resuscitate decisions need to be discussed and communicated to others—for example, ambulance staff—to prevent the sad situation of inappropriate and failed resuscitation attempts. Supporting carers in bereavement is a key role of primary care, with planned visits, consultation alerts by tagging of notes, pre-emptive supportive care, and referral to local bereavement support groups.

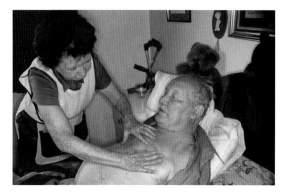

End of life care is important (reproduced with permission of Samuel Ashfield/Science Photo Library)

Other settings and patients without cancer

In assessing comprehensive palliative care services in a locality, other care settings must be considered. About 20% of people die in care homes and the end of life care provided for such people is important, though sometimes of variable quality. There are specific issues about care homes, such as their independent ownership, clinical governance, staff needs, multiple pathology of these patients, variable primary care arrangements, etc, which make this issue complex, and, despite best efforts, too often patients may be given suboptimal care and admitted to hospital in the final stages. Some care homes develop educational initiatives and specialist inreach and local guidelines, such as the use of pathways and frameworks, but this is an issue requiring further work to produce a more consistent high quality standard of care. Patients in private hospitals and community hospitals can sometimes be excluded from generalist and specialist palliative care services and provision may be suboptimal. Practices and procedures need to be agreed with the relevant staff and authorities to maintain high quality care for dying patients, such as symptom guidance, referral criteria, accessing specialist drugs, and support, etc.

The current provision of palliative care services in the UK still largely favours patients with cancer. Meanwhile, those with other common end stage diagnoses such as heart failure, COPD, renal failure, neurological disease, and dementia, who have equally severe symptoms with similarly poor prognoses, may have reduced access to services or specialist advice, especially in the community—for example, lack of specialist support, Marie Curie or Macmillan nurses, reduced access to advice or equipment etc. "Do I have to have cancer to get this kind of care?" is a natural response from patients with non-malignant but equally serious conditions. The improvements in management for patients with cancer by community providers need to be transferred to patients with other conditions. As an approximation, each year every GP has about 20 patients who die, of whom about five have cancer, five to seven have organ failure such as heart failure or COPD, and six to seven have old age comorbidities, frailty, and dementia, with one to two sudden deaths. The less predictable trajectories of illness in the group with organ failure mean greater hospital involvement and more difficulty predicting the terminal stages and introducing supportive care. For all patients with end stage illnesses, irrespective of the diagnosis, it is still important to apply palliative care principles, to recognise deterioration, and to include such patients in service provision—for example, specialist advice on accurate assessment and control of symptoms, respite care, access to equipment, information transfer, and handover forms.

Care needs for different disease trajectories

Predictable trajectory—for example, for patients with cancer
- Family support
- Symptom control
- Continuity of relationship
- Life closure
- Adaptability to rapid changes

Erratic trajectory—for example, for patients with organ system failure, heart failure, COPD, renal failure
- Preplanning for urgent situations
- Life closure
- Prevention of exacerbations
- Decision making about benefits of low yield treatments
- Support at home
- Prepare family for "sudden death"

Long term gradual decline—for example, for patients with dementia and frailty
- Endurance
- Long term home care service and supervision
- Helping carer to find meaning
- Avoiding unnecessary lingering
- Keeping skin intact
- Finding moments of joy and meaning for the patient

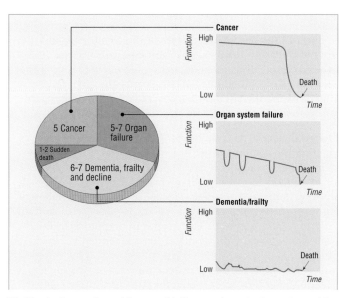

Workload of general practitioners, with illness trajectories for patients with cancer, organ failure, and old age, frailty, dementia, and decline

Multiprofessional teamwork

Specialist palliative care services, largely funded by the voluntary sector, have enhanced the quality of care given to dying patients throughout the world and improved our level of knowledge and understanding of the art and science of palliative care. The multiprofessional specialist palliative care team adds expertise and support to the generalist professionals in the community and to the patient and carer. Such support includes hospice outreach and hospice at home, respite admissions, clinical nurse specialists or Macmillan nurses, Marie Curie nurses providing hands-on nursing in patients' houses often overnight in the last days of life, day centres offering social support and activities and also complementary therapies, and much more.

Clinical challenges

Control of symptoms, particularly pain management, can be difficult in the community and is often poor, and better assessment, use of guidelines, and coworking with specialists can improve this. Education must be targeted and accessible and should include care of non-malignant conditions. For those in primary care, there may be some clinical conditions they rarely meet and may feel less confident to manage. Seeking specialist advice and reassurance that the best care is being provided can be invaluable, while maintaining the continuity of relationship provided by the primary care team. Some drugs often used in palliative care are not specifically licensed for that use and may be unfamiliar to GPs, so advice should be sought.

For many patients, including those with diagnoses other than cancer, development of "self care" and maximising of internal resources can be helpful, and the use of psychological or psycho-oncology services can help people to cope better.

Legal issues

The responsibility for notifying a death to the registrar lies with the relative or other person present at the death. A doctor who attended the patient during the last illness will normally issue a death certificate or report the case to the coroner. In the light of the Shipman inquiry, however, these procedures are currently being re-examined and some radical changes made. For more details consult the BMA website on www.bma.org.uk or your local primary care organisation.

Optimising home care—some models of good practice

So how can the best quality of care in the community and the best collaboration between generalist and specialists be ensured? Two complementary models are in current use in the UK to improve community palliative care—the gold standards framework for the last months/year of life and the Liverpool care pathway for the dying used in the last days of life.

The gold standards framework (GSF)

The GSF is a common sense, primary care based approach to formalising best practice, so that good care becomes standard for *all* patients *every* time. GSF users find it affirms their good practice, improves consistency of care so that "fewer patients slip through the net," and improves the experience of care for patients, carers, and staff. This work is underpinned by best available evidence, fully evaluated (recommended in NICE Guidance and by the Royal College of General Practitioners), and is extensively used by primary care teams across the UK.

The framework is easily used for patients without cancer nearing the end of life, and adaptations are developing for care homes, hospitals, and other settings.

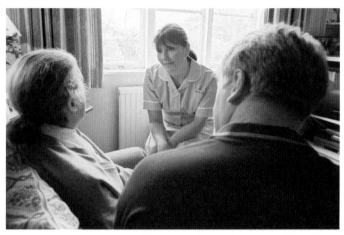

Marie Curie nurses provide hands-on care within the patient's home during the last days of life (with permission of Marie Curie Cancer Care)

The gold standards framework

The gold standards framework aims to develop a practice based system to improve and optimise the organisation and quality of care for patients and their carers in their last year of life. It can be summarised as follows:
- *One* gold standard for all patients nearing the end of life
- *Three* processes: identify, assess, and plan
- *Five* goals of the gold standard to enable patients to die well:
  Symptoms controlled as much as possible
  Living and dying where they choose
  Better advanced care planning information, feeling safe and supported with fewer crises
  Carers feeling supported, involved, empowered, and satisfied with care
  Staff feeling confident, satisfied with good communication, and team working with specialists
- *Seven* key tasks—the seven Cs:
  Communication
  Coordination
  Control of symptoms
  Continuity and out of hours
  Continued learning
  Cover support
  Care in the dying phase

For more details and resources, see www.goldstandardsframework.nhs.uk

---

The three central processes of GSF all involve improved communication
- *Identify* the key group of patients—for instance, using a register and agreed criteria
- *Assess* their main needs, both physical and psychosocial, and those of the carers
- *Plan* ahead for problems, including out of hours—move from *reactive* to *proactive* care by anticipation and prevention

The Liverpool care pathway (LCP)

The LCP was developed as a framework to enable generalist staff on hospital wards to care better for uncomplicated dying patients and later extended to the community, care homes, and hospice. An abbreviated form is integrated into the GSF as "C7." It allows standardisation and benchmarking of care to ensure consistency of care in the last few days of life. It is recommended that new areas in the community begin with GSF but later add LCP, while hospices and hospitals use LCP first.

Within England, the NHS Modernisation Agency and more recently the NHS End of Life Care Programme (www.modern.nhs.uk/cancer/endoflife) support these two established models of generalist care for patients with and without cancer. Advanced care planning tools are also recommended to promote choice and early planning discussions with patients, communicate decisions to others via a patient held record, and ensure more care focused on the patient. One example is the preferred place of care document that is in the early stages of use in England. Together, it is hoped that use of these tools will enable a better quality of palliative care to become mainstream within the NHS, with the "skilling up" of generalists, with fewer hospital admissions and more patients being enabled to die where they choose.

Conclusion

Good home care is vital. We now have the new situation of a population growing old and unwell more slowly than in previous generations—this is a new "epidemic" that we have not previously met or dealt with. With the demographic changes of ageing populations, better treatments and chronicity of end stage illnesses, fewer inpatient beds, and rising costs, there is a growing imperative to provide good home care for all seriously ill patients. Key issues include enablement of generalists, advanced care planning to determine need and preference, application of successful developments to patients with diseases other than cancer and in other settings, enhanced carer support and self care, high quality 24 hour clinical management and service provision, and good communication across boundaries.

As we rethink our palliative and supportive care services in response to this burgeoning need, the holistic approach of primary care is well placed to meet the challenge, if it is enabled to do so. Primary care teams in the community can deliver excellent palliative care for their dying patients and enable patients to die well where they choose when complemented by good access to specialist services, support, and expertise. As demand for community care increases in future, it is important to maximise the potential of primary palliative care and the use of frameworks or protocols with good collaboration with specialists.

Best practice in the last hours and days of life

(See for example, the Liverpool care pathway, www.lcp-mariecurie.org.uk)
- Current medications are assessed and non-essentials discontinued
- "As required" subcutaneous medication is prescribed according to an agreed protocol to manage pain, agitation, nausea and vomiting, and respiratory tract secretions
- Decisions are taken to discontinue inappropriate interventions, including blood tests, intravenous fluids, and observation of vital signs
- The insights of the patient, family, and carers into the patient's condition are identified
- Religious and spiritual needs of the patient, family, and carers are assessed
- Means of informing family and carers of the patient's impending death are identified
- The family and carers are given appropriate written information
- The GP's practice is made aware of the patient's condition
- A plan of care is explained and discussed with the patient, family, and carers

A death dominated by fear, crises, inappropriate admissions, overmedicalisation, and poor communication can be a tragedy and a failure of our medical system; enabling a peaceful death at home can be a great accomplishment for all concerned

Further reading
- Gomas J-M. Palliative care at home: A reality or mission impossible? *Pall Med* 1993;7:45–59.
- Piercy J. The plight of the informal carer. In: Charlton R, ed. *Primary palliative care*. Oxford: Radcliffe Medical Press, 2002.
- Simon C. Informal carers and the primary care team. *Br J Gen Pract* 2001;51:920–3.
- Thomas K. Out of hours palliative care—bridging the gap. *Eur J Pall Care* 2000;7:22–5.

17 Bereavement

Marilyn Relf

Bereavement is a universal human experience. The way it is experienced and expressed varies, reflecting such factors as the meaning of the lost relationship, personality, and ways of coping. The loss of an important relationship is a personal crisis, and, like other stressful life events, bereavement has serious health consequences for a substantial minority of people. It is associated with high mortality for some groups and up to a third of bereaved people develop a depressive illness. Help targeted at those most at risk has been shown to be effective and to make the most efficient use of scarce resources.

Grief

Grief is multidimensional. It has an impact on behaviour, emotions, cognitive processes, physical health, social functioning, and spiritual beliefs. A major loss forces people to adapt their assumptions about the world and about themselves, and grief is a transitional process by which people assimilate the reality of their loss and find a way of living without the external presence of the person who died. Traditionally, this process has been described as consisting of overlapping phases. While it is more useful to think of grief as characterised by simultaneous change and adjustment, such models provide useful descriptions of the major themes of grief.

The initial reaction is shock and disbelief accompanied by a sense of unreality. This occurs even when death is expected but may last longer and be more intense after an unexpected loss.

Numbness is replaced with waves of intense pining and distress. The desire to recover a loved one is strong and preoccupation with memories, restless searching, dreams, and auditory and sensory awareness of the deceased are common. Bereavement affects the immune system, and physical symptoms may also be caused by anxiety and changes in behaviour such as loss of sleep or altered nutrition, or may mimic the symptoms of the deceased. A crucial factor is the meaning of the loss, and bereaved people search for an understanding of why and how the death occurred. The events surrounding the death may be obsessively reviewed. For some, there may be questioning of previously deeply held beliefs, while others find great support from their faith, the rituals associated with it, and the social contact with others that religious affiliation often brings. Symptoms of depression such as despair, poor concentration, apathy, social withdrawal, lack of purpose, and sadness are common for more than a year after an important bereavement. This reflects the multidimensional impact of loss.

To carry on without what they have lost, bereaved people may need to rebuild their identities, find new purpose, acquire new skills, and take on new roles. Gradually people manage these adjustments more effectively and more positive feelings emerge accompanied by renewed energy and hope for the future. Eventually most bereaved people can remember the deceased without feeling overwhelmed. The deceased continue to be part of their lives, however, and family events and anniversaries may reawaken painful memories and feelings. In this sense there is no definite end point that marks "recovery" from grief.

A central notion of traditional models of grief is that it must be confronted and expressed, otherwise it may manifest in some other way, such as depression or anxiety. Throughout the period of mourning, however, most people cope by oscillating

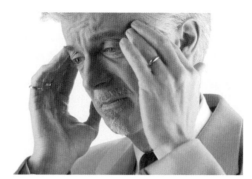

Courtesy of photos.com

Dimensions of loss and common expressions of grief

Dimension	Expression
Emotions	
Depression	Episodic waves of dejection, sadness, sorrow, despair
Anxiety	Fear of breaking down, going crazy, dying, not coping
Guilt	About events surrounding loss or past behaviour
Anger	Anger/irritation with deceased, family, professionals, God
Loneliness	Feeling alone, bouts of intense loneliness
Loss of enjoyment	Nothing can be pleasurable without the deceased
Relief	Relief now the suffering of the deceased has ended
Behaviours	
Agitation	Tension, restlessness, overactivity, searching for deceased
Fatigue	Cognitive impairment, lassitude, poor concentration
Crying	Tears, sad expression
Attitudes	
Self reproach	Regrets about past behaviour toward deceased
Low self esteem	Inadequacy, failure, incompetence, worthlessness
Hopelessness	Loss of purpose, apathy, no desire to go on living
Sense of unreality	Feeling removed from current events
Suspicion	Doubting others
Social withdrawal	Difficulty in maintaining relationships
Toward deceased	Yearning/pining, preoccupation, hallucinations, idealisation
Physiological	
Appetite	Loss of appetite, weight change
Sleep	Insomnia, early morning waking
Physical complaints	Such as, headaches, muscular pains, indigestion, shortness of breath, blurred vision, lump in throat, sighing, dry mouth, palpitations, hair loss
Substance use	Increased use of psychotropic medicines, alcohol, tobacco
Illness	Particularly infections and stress related illness
Spiritual	
Search for meaning and purpose	Questioning beliefs and purpose of life. Finding comfort in faith, beliefs, rituals
Identity	
Identity	Changes to self concept, self esteem

between confronting grief (for example, thinking about the deceased, pining, holding on to memories, expressing feelings) and seeking distraction to manage everyday life (for example, suppressing memories and taking "time off" from grief by keeping busy, regulating emotions). Neither pattern of coping is problematic and difficulties are likely only if the balance of behaviour is oriented exclusively on loss (chronic grief) or avoidance (absent grief). Although grief is universal, social norms vary and what is viewed as "normal" differs both within and across cultures. Personality factors, sex, and cultural background will influence the degree of individual oscillation—for example, women may be more emotional and loss focused while men may be more inclined to cope by seeking information, thinking through problems, taking action, and seeking diversion.

Factors associated with poor adjustment

Research has identified several factors that influence the course of grief and are associated with ongoing poor health. There are three groups of factors: situational, individual, and environmental.

Situational is the circumstances surrounding the death and the impact of concurrent life events. Deaths that are untimely, unexpected, stigmatised, or unduly disturbing cause more severe and more prolonged grief. The death of someone with terminal illness can still be unexpected and distressing, and the strain of caring for a terminally ill person for more than six months also increases risk. People from minority cultural or ethnic groups may experience problems if they are not able to follow the rituals and customs they think are appropriate. Concurrent crises such as multiple losses and financial difficulties also strain coping resources.

Individual factors concern the meaning of the lost relationship and personal factors. The subjective meaning of the loss is more important than kinship, and the closer the relationship, the greater the risk. The more necessary the deceased was for the bereaved person's sense of wellbeing and self esteem, the more all pervading the sense of loss. The loss of a child is particularly difficult. Highly ambivalent relationships are associated with continuing high levels of distress, particularly guilt. Studies that compare the health of widows and widowers with married people show that widowers are at greater risk, particularly younger men. Pre-existing health problems may be exacerbated by bereavement, and the risk of suicide is greater among those who have had a previous psychiatric illness.

Environmental is the social and cultural context of risk. A perceived lack of support is the common factor. Bereavement may deprive people of their main source of support and shared suffering, and differential grieving patterns within social networks may compound this. Family discord is a source of additional stress. Among elderly people, poor health, reduced mobility, and sensory losses may make it more difficult to cope and reduce the capacity to develop new interests or relationships.

Assessing complicated grief

As grief and its expression are influenced by the society in which a bereaved individual lives, and by attitudes and expectations in the immediate family, assessing grief is complex. The focus should be on understanding the individual and on recognising their strengths and resources as well as potential difficulties. The following should be taken into account:

Intensity and duration of feelings and behaviour—A woman who cries every day in the first few weeks after the loss of her husband or partner is within the normal range; if she is doing

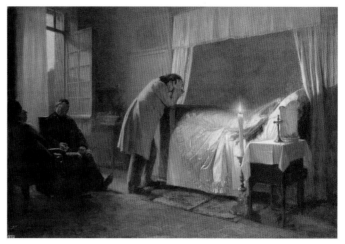

"The death of Madame Bovary" by Albert-Auguste Fourie (b 1854). Reproduced with permission from Musée des Beaux-Arts, Rouen, France/ Lauros / Giraudon/ The Bridgeman Art Library

---

Factors to consider when assessing risk

Situational
- How distressing was the illness and death?
- Concurrent stress

Individual
- Meaning and nature of the lost relationship
- Previous physical and psychological health
- Personality and coping style

Social
- Quality of support

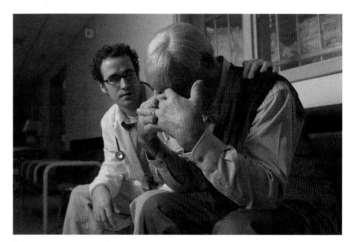

A bereavement can take away a person's main source of support (photos.com)

so 12 months later there is cause for concern. Prolonged intense pining, self reproach, and anger are danger signals, as is prolonged withdrawal from social contact. Failure to show any grief may also be problematic, but people cope in different ways and some recover quickly, especially if they were well prepared for the death.

Culturally determined mourning practices—A mother who maintains the room of her young son, who died four years ago, as a shrine would be unusual in the UK. In Japan, however, a widow might talk to her dead husband for the rest of her life as she makes offerings at the household shrine. In the UK, the norm is to keep feelings private, and men in particular may experience social pressure to suppress emotion.

Risk factors described above that may make grief more intense and prolonged.

Personality—It is important to understand how individuals usually cope with challenges. Do they normally express emotion dramatically or are they self contained and private? How characteristic is the behaviour? What aspects of their situation are particularly distressing for them?

Vulnerable groups

Children

Well meaning adults often wish to protect children from painful events but by doing so often leave children feeling excluded from events that are important to them. Children begin to develop an understanding of some aspects of death and bereavement as early as 2 or 3 years. By the age of 5, over half of children have full understanding, and virtually all children will by the age of 8. How early a child develops such understanding depends primarily on whether adults have given truthful and sensitive explanations of any experiences of loss that the child may have had, such as the death of pets, and only secondarily on the level of cognitive development.

When a death is about to occur, or has occurred, it is helpful to discuss with parents what experience of death their children have and what they have been told, and understand, about the current situation. It is important to encourage children to ask questions. Parents are the best people to talk to their children, but they may need support and advice from professionals. Families often find it helpful to create memory boxes to store treasured photos and keepsakes, to read storybooks, or to use the workbooks on death and bereavement that are now available.

Parents may be preoccupied with the practical challenges of caring for someone who is dying or overwhelmed with their own grief. It may be useful to involve family friends or teachers. Adolescents struggling to develop their individuality and independence may find members of their peer group to be helpful, particularly if they know someone who has also experienced bereavement.

Support and information is available from national and local organisations concerned with the needs of children experiencing bereavement.

Confused elderly people and those with learning difficulties

The needs of these groups for help in dealing with bereavement have often been ignored. Repeated explanations and supported involvement in the important events, such as the funeral and visiting the grave, have been shown to reduce the repetitious questions about the whereabouts of the dead person by confused elderly people or difficult and withdrawn behaviour in people with learning disabilities. This makes their continuing care less demanding for both family and professional groups.

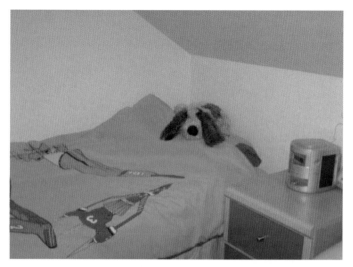

It would be unusual in the UK for a mother to maintain the room of a dead child as a shrine

---

Books for children to read or use

- Varley S. *Badger's parting gifts*. London: Pictures Lions, 1994. Available in other languages.
- Crossley D. *Muddles, puddles and sunshine*. Gloucester: Winston's Wish, 2000.
- Couldrick A. *When your mum or dad has cancer*. Oxford: Sobell Publications, 1991.
- Heegard M. *When someone very special dies*. Minneapolis: Woodland Press, 1988. (Workbook)
- Stickney D. *Waterbugs and dragonflies*. London: Mowbray, 1982.

Organisations such as Winston's Wish and the Child Bereavement Trust offer a wide range of publications and resources for children and their families

---

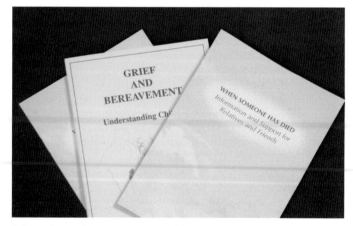

Information on bereavement is available from a number of sources — local and national

What helps?

Identifying people whose grief may be more complex—Many difficulties can be avoided by work before the death to minimise the effect of factors that increase the risks to health and wellbeing associated with bereavement. It is helpful to involve family members in decision making, provide information, check out what people understand, encourage questions, and offer opportunities after bereavement to talk to those who provided care at the end of life. If misunderstandings or disagreements about the care of the patient are ignored, family members may remain angry and distressed and find it harder to make sense of their situation.

Being present at the death, seeing the body afterwards, and attending funerals and memorial services—These are helpful provided the bereaved person wishes to participate. It may be the first time an adult has seen a dead person, and information should be given about what to expect. Children and young people should be offered the choice to see the body and attend funerals provided they are given appropriate explanations about what to expect and support.

Providing information—Information about how to register a death, common aspects of grief, and local and national support services should be provided through empathetic personal contact and easy to read leaflets.

Bereavement support and counselling—While grief is a normal reaction to loss, the general lack of understanding combined with social pressure to keep feelings private means that bereaved people may feel isolated and find it hard to seek help. One advantage of palliative care is that support can be offered to bereaved people without them having to seek help. Therapeutic counselling is unlikely to be needed by most bereaved people. A substantial minority, however, benefit from services that provide sensitive listening, reassurance, and help with managing all the changes posed by bereavement. It is good practice to assess the need for ongoing support and to offer support proactively, particularly to those who lack social support, where the events surrounding the death have been particularly distressing, or whose history or personality may increase the risk of prolonged grief. It is also important to give information about how to access bereavement services to those who are not being contacted proactively. Support from volunteers, provided with training, supervision, and back up from suitably qualified professionals, has been shown to reduce the use of general practitioners' services. Counselling to unselected groups shows little benefit.

Opportunities to meet other bereaved people—Informal social events or more formal groups enable bereaved people to safely test out the often disturbing feelings, questions, and thoughts that they have with others facing similar circumstances.

There is no single intervention that meets the needs of all bereaved people, but there is an increasing range of resources for them to draw on. Most hospices offer bereavement services. Individual and telephone support provided by volunteers is the main support strategy but groups and memorial services are also common. Many areas have branches of national self help organisations. In addition counsellors, psychologists, social workers, and community psychiatric nurses have the skills to work with the minority of bereaved people whose grief is more complicated by their personality or history of psychological or social problems.

Useful organisations

Childhood Bereavement Network
8 Wakley Street, London EC1V 7QE (tel 020 7843 6309)
A national network of service providers. Contact for information about resources for bereaved children

Child Bereavement Trust
Aston House, High Street, West Wycombe, Bucks HP14 3AG (tel 01494 446648, helpline 0845 357 1000)
www.childbereavement.org.uk
Resources and information for bereaved families and for professionals

Child Death Helpline
Bereavement Services Department, Great Ormond Street Hospital, Great Ormond Street, London WC1N 3JH (tel 020 7813 8551, helpline: 0800 282986)
Befriending and emotional support from volunteer bereaved parents for those affected by the death of a child

Compassionate Friends
53 North Street, Bristol BS3 1EN (tel 0117 966 5202, helpline 0845 123 2304) www.tcf.org.uk
National organisation with local branches. Offers befriending to bereaved parents after loss of child of any age

Cruse Bereavement Care
Cruse House, 126 Sheen Road, Richmond TW9 1UR (tel 020 8939 9530, helpline 0870 167 1677) www.crusebereavement.org.uk
National organisation with local branches. Offers bereavement support, counselling, advice, and information

Jewish Bereavement Counselling Service
8–10 Forty Avenue, Wembley, Middlesex (tel 020 8385 1874)
www.jvisit.org.uk
Counselling by trained volunteers. Telephone helpline

Lesbian and Gay Bereavement Project
Healthy Gay Living Centre, 40 Borough High Street, London SE1 1XW (tel 020 7403 5969 restricted hours)
Trained volunteers offer support and information to bereaved lesbians and gay men and their families and friends; education; telephone helpline (evenings)

SANDS (Stillbirth and Neonatal Death Society)
28 Portland Place, London W1B 1LY (tel 020 7436 7940, helpline 020 7436 5881)
Support for parents after stillbirth or neonatal death

Winston's Wish
Clara Burgess Centre, Bayshill Road, Cheltenham GL50 3AW (tel 01242 515157, helpline 0845 20 30 40 5) www.winstonswish.org.uk
Offers a range of services for bereaved children and young people including national helpline, information for family members, resources, publications, and training for professionals

Further reading

- Abrams R. *When parents die.* London: Routledge, 1999.
- Blackman N. *Loss and learning disability.* London: Worth Publishing, 2003.
- Couldrick A. *Grief and bereavement: understanding children.* Oxford: Sobell House Publications, 1988.
- Dyregrov A. *Grief in children.* London: Jessica Kingsley, 1990.
- Klass D, Silverman PR, Nickman SL. *Continuing bonds.* Washington: Taylor and Francis, 1996.
- Martin TL, Doka KJ. *Men don't cry . . . women do.* Philadelphia: Taylor and Francis, 2000.
- Parkes CM, Laungani P, Young B. *Death and bereavement across cultures.* London: Routledge, 1997.
- Parkes CM, Relf M, Couldrick A. *Counselling in terminal care and bereavement.* Leicester: BPS Books, 1996.
- Payne S, Horn S, Relf M. *Loss and bereavement.* Buckingham: Open University Press, 1999.
- Stroebe MS, Stroebe W, Hansson RO. *Handbook of bereavement: theory, research and intervention.* Cambridge: Cambridge University Press, 1993.

18 Complementary therapies

Michelle Kohn, Jane Maher

Definition of terms

In the past complementary therapies were described as "unconventional therapies" rarely used by orthodox medical professionals. Now, with increased use and understanding of these therapies, the term "complementary" has been adopted to indicate therapies that can work alongside and in conjunction with orthodox medical treatment. The term "integrated health care" is also used to describe the provision of orthodox and complementary treatments side by side as a package of care.

The term "alternative therapies" indicates therapies used instead of orthodox medical treatments (BMA, 1993). In the US, the former office of alternative medicine of the National Institutes of Health coined the term "complementary and alternative medicine," or CAM, to encompass both approaches. This term includes a much broader spectrum of medical and therapeutic approaches to those used in palliative care.

In the context of palliative care, we have used the term "complementary" to refer to those therapies that are used alongside conventional health care.

Classification

Therapies can be classified in various ways. They may be grouped by whether they have a direct physical application (such as massage), a primarily psychological effect (such as visualisation), or whether they purport to have a pharmacological basis (such as dietary supplements). They can also be classified by application—that is, they can be thought of as a complete system of care (such as homoeopathy), as useful techniques (such as aromatherapy), or as approaches to self help (such as meditation). More recently, the House of Lords select committee report provided a classification, grouping therapies according to their professional regulation and evidence base.

In palliative care, patterns of provision vary widely. Therapies may be offered by individual practitioners based in the hospital or community or in a designated setting where several practitioners offer a wider range of therapies with a more comprehensive package of care. This may be within a hospital or hospice or in a separate location often set up by voluntary organisations or self help and support groups.

Patterns of use

The use of complementary therapies in palliative care is considerable and growing. Use by adults with cancer has been estimated as between 7% and 64%. Users are likely to be younger, female, and have higher education levels, income, and social class. Use is also associated with progression of the disease, attendance at support groups, and previous use.

Provision of therapies is mainly in hospices and hospitals. Those most commonly on offer to patients are:

- Touch therapies, such as aromatherapy, reflexology, and massage
- Mind-body therapies such as relaxation and visualisation
- Acupuncture
- Healing and energy work, such as reiki, spiritual healing, and therapeutic touch
- Nutritional and medicinal therapies, such as vitamins and dietary supplements, homoeopathy, and herbal remedies.

Disciplines in complementary and alternative medicine (as grouped by the House of Lords Science and Technology Select Committee 6th Report, November 2000)

Group 1—professionally organised alternative therapies	Group 2—complementary therapies	Group 3—alternative disciplines
Acupuncture* Chiropractic Herbal medicine (includes essiac*) Homoeopathy* Osteopathy	Alexander technique Aromatherapy* Bach and other flower remedies Bodywork therapies including massage* Counselling stress therapy* Hypnotherapy* Reflexology* Meditation* Shiatsu* Healing* Marharishi ayurvedic medicine Nutritional medicine* Yoga*	3a: Long established traditional systems of health care Anthroposophical medicine (includes iscador*) Ayurvedic medicine Chinese herbal medicine* Eastern medicine Traditional Chinese medicine Naturopathy medicine 3b: Other alternative disciplines Crystal therapy Dowsing Iridology Kinesiology

*Therapies commonly used in palliative care.

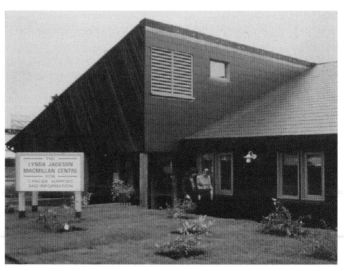

The Lynda Jackson Macmillan Centre at the Mount Vernon Cancer Centre provides a drop-in information and support service. Appointments can be made for complementary therapies, counselling, relaxation sessions, educational sessions, and advice on benefits (photo reproduced with permission)

These services are often extended to both carers and staff and, encouragingly, most are free of charge.

The role of complementary therapies
The role of complementary therapies in palliative care is presently undefined. Three basic models of how therapies might be used have been proposed. These are the

- Humanistic model, where the aim is to provide a supportive role by relieving symptoms, side effects of treatment, and improving quality of life
- Holistic model, where the aim is to empower the user by giving patients greater control over their health and quality of life
- Radical holistic model, where self healing is the proposed aim and patients seek increased survival and possible cure.

Considerable overlap may exist between the models—for example, patients may be given a treatment as a support and find it empowering. The radical model is usually advocated outside the NHS setting as an alternative to orthodox treatment.

Why do patients seek complementary therapies?

Knowing why patients seek therapies is fundamental in evaluating their use. Possible factors "pushing" patients away from orthodox medicine and those "pulling" them towards complementary therapies can be identified. The provision of "touch, talk, and time" and a "healing" environment seem to be particularly important.

In 2002 the Department of Health commissioned further research into the use of therapies from diagnosis through to palliative and terminal care. Drivers for use, perceived benefits, and comparisons with orthodox medical care are also being evaluated.

Referral and assessment

Referral
Patients and carers should be able to self refer or have a family member or health professional refer them for assessment for complementary therapies.

All healthcare professionals working in palliative care are advised to be familiar with complementary therapies and, when appropriate, refer patients to further sources of information and services. Referral criteria are useful if health professionals are making referrals. They may also help to guide patients when they are self referring. When possible, it is recommended that there is a designated facilitator or coordinator to ensure continuity of care and to offer patients information to make their own informed choice of treatment.

Assessment
The assessment
Assessment ranges in different settings from screening for contraindications to a full assessment of physical, psychological, emotional, and spiritual factors affecting the patient. Contraindications and precautions for use of individual therapies should also be discussed.

Contraindications and precautions
Many questions arise in the treatment of patients with serious illness and widespread disease. For example, a question often asked, and an issue where confusion arises, is whether massage spreads cancer. Based on current evidence, cancer is not a contraindication to receiving gentle massage, though massage therapists are advised to be cautious over tumour sites.

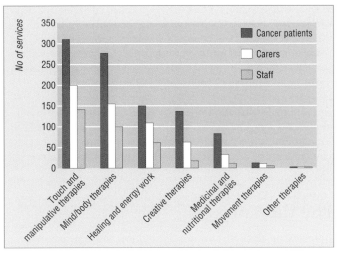

Number of services in the UK offering various complementary therapies to patients with cancer, their carers, and staff (Macmillan Directory 2002)

Why do people use/want complementary therapies?

Orthodox medicine—"push" factors:
- Failure to produce curative treatments
- Adverse effects of orthodox medicine—for example, side effects of chemotherapy
- Lack of time with practitioner, loss of bedside skills
- Dissatisfaction with the technical approach
- Fragmentation of care due to specialization

Complementary therapies—"pull" factors:
- Media reports of dramatic improvements produced by complementary therapies
- Belief that complementary therapies are natural
- Empowerment of patient through lifestyle and psychological equilibrium
- Focus on spiritual and emotional wellbeing
- Provision by therapist of "touch, talk, and time"
- Provision of a non-clinical "healing" environment

Criteria for referral based on current evidence
- Relaxation
- To improve quality of life and wellbeing
- For support
- Tension, stress
- Anxiety, fear, panic attacks
- Low mood, depression
- Fatigue
- Insomnia
- Pain
- Breathlessness
- Nausea and vomiting
- Constipation
- Hot flushes
- Muscular skeletal problems
- Altered body image

Discussion should include:
- What the therapies are
- What they mean
- What is involved in the treatment
- What side effects might occur
- What outcome can be hoped for

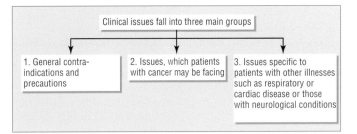

Contraindications to use of complementary therapies

Deep massage to any part of the body is not advisable for those with active cancer to avoid trauma and activation of the immune response. The National Guidelines for the Use of Complementary Therapies in Supportive and Palliative Care (produced by the Prince of Wales's Foundation for Integrated Health and National Council for Hospice and Specialist Palliative Care Services) detail contraindications and precautions for the therapies most used in palliative care, in addition to a wealth of information relevant to those setting up or maintaining services. Issues such as development and management of the service, practice development, and the evidence base for therapies are examined.

The therapies

The table on page 81 outlines those therapies most commonly used by patients in palliative care. The list is not exhaustive and excludes the more peripheral therapies—for example, crystal therapy. The choice of therapies depends on what the patient hopes to gain. Some may prefer to learn a relaxation technique to have a tool for further self care, some may enjoy a yoga class with the camaraderie of a group activity, and others might enjoy a more passive "one on one" approach and select a touch therapy such as aromatherapy.

Types of evidence

Although the scientific evidence for complementary therapies is sparse, this does not mean they are ineffective. Rather it reflects the limited resources that have been committed to research and that many clinical trials have been of poor methodological quality. The factors that have hindered research into the effectiveness of complementary therapies are well documented, as are the difficulties of conducting research on people with a life threatening condition or advanced and progressive illness.

Evidence has been gathered from randomised controlled trials, prospective studies with a comparison group, comparison group studies, cross sectional studies, professional consensus, and anecdotes from patients. It is clear from numerous surveys and service evaluations that patients do value complementary therapies as an integral part of their care. More research from various perspectives and methodological approaches is needed.

Evaluating complementary therapies

Although the randomised controlled trial is the method of choice for evaluating a simple intervention, it may be inappropriate for researching certain complex therapies as the non-specific effects may be integral to the therapies rather than a confounding factor. Where randomisation is involved, there is evidence that "non-specific effects" are reduced if the intervention is not thought to be effective, either by the practitioner or the patient. Finding an appropriate placebo is challenging for many of these interventions—for example, using a "control" for massage.

In designing trials, methodologists need a clear objective of what the trial aims to achieve—appropriate questions must be asked, which depend on shared language and understanding the nature of the therapy. Defining realistic outcomes and using appropriate measuring tools are key in achieving results. For example, patients may still experience pain but feel better able to cope. Thus symptoms alone may miss the perceived value of the intervention. There may also be additional benefits, such as enjoying a greater sense of "wellness," which traditional outcome measures might miss. Study design should appropriately reflect the benefits expressed by patients, using a mixture of qualitative and quantitative methods.

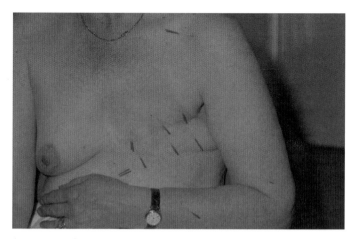

Acupuncture for pain around mastectomy scar

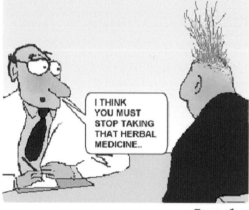

I THINK YOU MUST STOP TAKING THAT HERBAL MEDICINE..

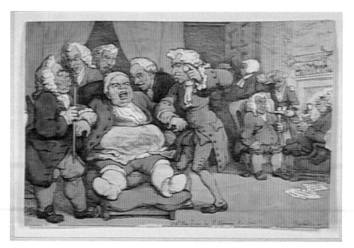

A therapeutic relationship? "The consultation, or last hope" by Thomas Rowlandson, 1808. Reproduced from Emery A, Emery M. *Medicine and art.* RSM Press: London, 2002

The two cartoons in this chapter are courtesy of Quack.

Complementary therapies

Touch therapies

Aromatherapy
Many plant species contain essential oils, which give them their distinctive smell. These oils can be condensed by a distillation process to create a concentrated aromatic solution. Practitioners believe that essential oils can have particular physiological or psychological effects

Reflexology
Reflexology has its roots in traditional Chinese medicine. Practitioners apply pressure to specific zones on the soles and tops of the feet to assess the disease state of the patient and also to improve health. Massaging the points is thought to unblock energy pathways and restore normal energy flow

Massage
Massage is a generic term for various techniques that involve touching, pressing, or kneading the surfaces of the body to promote mental and physical relaxation

The evidence base for use of the touch therapies is growing. A wide range of uses includes helping to promote relaxation, alleviate anxiety, reduce depression, reduce pain, reduce nausea, alleviate symptoms such as breathlessness, alleviate side effects of chemotherapy, improve sleep pattern, reduce stress and tension, reduce psychological distress, provide emotional support, improve wellbeing and quality of life, encourage acceptance of altered body image

Nutritional and medicinal

Herbal remedies
Plant products have been used for centuries and many Western allopathic medicines, including oncology drugs, are derived from plants. Plants contain many potentially effective compounds and determining which are beneficial and which are harmful is a challenge. Moreover, the constituents may work synergistically to provide the effects

Homoeopathy
Homoeopathy is based on the ancient principle that "like can treat like." Homoeopathic remedies are prepared from a mother tincture, which is diluted down in successive steps. At each step the solution is given a vigorous shake, and homoeopaths believe that the power of the diluted solution to heal is conferred during these successive shakes.

Hundreds of herbal remedies are purported to have benefits in palliative care, including anticancer benefits as well as more general immune enhancing effects. Most of them do not have proven specific benefits but this could be due to the quality of the trials conducted. Possible interactions with active treatment and side effects necessitate caution in recommending their use. Careful discussion with a knowledgeable health professional is recommended. The evidence of clinical effectiveness of homoeopathy is mixed and scientific research into homoeopathy in cancer is in its infancy. Nevertheless, homoeopathy is used by patients in palliative care, and there is evidence that they find the approach helpful. The best available evidence suggests effectiveness of use for fatigue, hot flushes, pain including joint pain and muscle spasm, anxiety and stress, depression, quality of life including mood disturbance, radiotherapy, skin reactions, and ileus after surgery

Healing and energy work

Reiki
Reiki is a method of healing that was rediscovered in Japan in the 1800s. The energy is known as qi and can be channelled from its originating source by the reiki practitioner and passed on to a recipient

Spiritual healing
Spiritual healing, often referred to simply as healing, involves channeling of healing energies through the healer to the patient. It is a supportive approach, which may involve light touch or no touch at all, depending on the recipient's conditions and wishes

The best available evidence suggests that reiki and spiritual healing may contribute to pain relief, promote relaxation, to improve sleep patterns, reduce tension, stress and anxiety, to provide emotional and/or spiritual support, contribute to a sense of wellbeing, reduce side effects of chemotherapy and radiotherapy, and support the patient in the dying process

Mind-body therapies

Hypnotherapy/hypnosis
The aim of these therapies is to alter the quality of an individual's thoughts and thought processes. This could lead to psychological and possibly physiological change. As well as simple relaxation there is classical meditation involving various techniques

Visualisation
Patients are said to be able to overcome physical and emotional problems by imagining positive images and desired outcomes to specific situations, either alone or helped by a practitioner in a process known as guided imagery

A large body of evidence exists for the use of clinical hypnosis in supportive and palliative care. It may be useful to enhance the immune response, as an adjunct to more conventional forms of psychotherapy, to enhance coping ability, to enhance recovery from surgery, to reduce nausea related to chemotherapy, to increase tolerance of scanning and radiotherapy procedures, to reduce pain, in mood disturbance and emotional and psychological distress, to enhance quality of life, to reduce anxiety and depression

Others

Acupuncture
Acupuncture has its roots in traditional Chinese medicine and is therefore part of a system involving multiple therapeutic interventions such as diet, manipulation, meditation, and herbal medicine. The aim is to restore the energy balance and health. The therapeutic technique involves the insertion of fine needles under the skin and underlying tissues at specific points for therapeutic or preventative purposes

Current evidence supports the use of acupuncture and acupressure in palliative care for the treatment of nausea and vomiting induced by chemotherapy and after surgery, with high level evidence emerging for acute pain and xerostomia. Despite limited scientific evidence, there are also data to support its use in palliative care for pain associated with diseases other than cancer, breathlessness, radiation induced rectitis, hiccups, hot flushes, angina, and AIDS

Regulation and training of therapists

Many health professionals are choosing to train as complementary therapists. They most commonly train in acupuncture and the touch therapies. Many complementary therapists, however, do not have any biomedical training beyond their therapies.

With the exception of osteopaths and chiropractors, who are regulated by law, most complementary therapy practice is either voluntarily self regulated or unregulated. In general, therapists recognise the need for self regulation, both to enhance their professional credibility and to protect the public. The therapies used mostly by patients in palliative care—aromatherapy, reflexology, and massage—are not statutorily regulated and are fragmented. Many of the complementary professions are working towards common standards of education and training and the accreditation of professional courses. In 2001 the Department of Health recommended that any accreditation board is completely independent of the institutions to be accredited.

The Qualifications and Curriculum Authority (QCA) in England provides details of external awarding bodies on its website (www.qca.org.uk).

Sources of information

Most research in the UK has focused on touch and mind-body therapies. Cancer organisations and charities have information on these therapies. There is little information available, however, on medicinal and nutritional approaches such as vitamin use and dietary supplements. Patients do use these products, often without the knowledge of their health professionals. Their use may be intended as complementary but the effects may not be. Further attention needs to be given to this issue with consideration of possible drug interactions and interference with orthodox treatment and educating patients to make informed decisions about their use.

There is an overwhelming amount of information available, much of which is inaccurate. Health professionals and patients wanting information about individual therapies and local resources are advised to consult reliable sources of information such as:

- The Research Council for Complementary Medicine—a CAM and cancer database is in development (sponsored by the DoH). This will be available both for professionals and patients with clinical appraisals for each therapy
- Websites/helplines/brochures from cancer organisations such as the NCRI, Cancerbackup, Cancer Research UK, or Macmillan Cancer Relief
- International websites—for example, the NIH's NCCAM and the NCI's OCCAM in the US
- Voluntary sector organisations and self help and support groups
- Health professionals such as general practitioners and Macmillan and Marie Curie nurses
- Local cancer units/centres and hospices
- Cancer information and support centres
- The National Institute for Clinical Excellence (NICE); as part of the Guidance on Cancer Services—Improving Supportive and Palliative Care for Adults with Cancer (2004), NICE have recommended that information on complementary therapy resources be made available for each local cancer network.

For the future, it is hoped that with appropriate sources of information and provision of services, backed up by appropriate research, complementary therapies will become an integral part of palliative care.

Do's and don'ts—a checklist for patients

Do . . .

- Establish what the therapy is intended to achieve
- Use a therapist who has a recognised qualification, belongs to a professional body, and has insurance. Ask if the person is experienced and/or trained in treating patients with your condition
- Ask for an informal chat with the therapist and/or for any leaflets or literature supplied by them
- Find out what the fees are (if any) and what these cover
- Talk to family, friends, and health professionals about your plans
- Consult any relevant fact sheets/telephone helplines provided by reputable support organisations for patients
- Find out what is available on the NHS, in treatment centres you may already be using or through your family doctor at the medical centre. Wherever you are, ask about the availability of the full range of complementary therapy services

Don't . . .

- Abandon proved conventional treatments
- Be misled by promises or suggestions of cures or respond to a "hard sell" that offers simple solutions
- Rely on a single source of information as it may be inaccurate
- Use a therapist who cannot refer you to the relevant research
- Feel pressured to buy expensive books, videos, nutritional supplements, or herbal preparations as part of a therapy
- Be afraid to ask for references and credentials
- Accept treatment from someone who makes you feel uncomfortable in any way

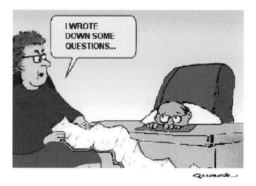

Other useful sources of information

Publications

- Kohn M. *Complementary therapies in cancer care—abridged report of a study produced for Macmillan Cancer Relief.* London: Macmillan Cancer Relief (UK), 1999.
- *Directory of complementary therapy services in UK cancer care.* London: Macmillan Cancer Relief (UK), 2002.
- *National guidelines for the use of complementary therapies in supportive and palliative care.* London: Prince of Wales's Foundation for Integrated Health, National Council for Hospice and Specialist Palliative Care Services, 2003.
- House of Lords Select Committee on Science and Technology. *Complementary and alternative medicine.* London: Stationery Office, 2000. (HL Paper 123)

Websites

- National Cancer Institute's Office of Cancer Complementary and Alternative Medicine (OCCAM), USA. www3.cancer.gov/occam
- National Center for Complementary and Alternative Medicine (NCCAM), at the National Institutes of Health, USA. http://nccam.nih.gov
- American Cancer Society. www.cancer.org/docroot/home/index.asp
- CancerHelp UK. www.cancerhelp.org.uk
- Macmillan Cancer Relief. www.macmillan.org.uk
- Bristol Cancer Help Centre. www.bristolcancerhelp.org
- National Cancer Research Institute (NCRI), Complementary Therapies Clinical Studies Development Group. www.ncri.org.uk
- The Prince's Foundation for Integrated Health. www.fihealth.org.uk

Index

Index

Index

Index